Tim Jainniney 11/5/00

WORKBOOK

BRADY

Being A Long-Term Care Nursing Assistant

Fourth Edition Update Grade - A

Connie A. Will-Black, RN, BSN
Judith B. Eighmy, RN, BSN

BRADY
PRENTICE HALL
Upper Saddle River, New Jersey 07458

Project manager: **Janet McGillicuddy/Julie Boddorf**
Acquisitions editor: **Barbara Krawiec**
Director of manufacturing and production: **Bruce Johnson**
Manufacturing buyer: **Ilene Sanford**
Editorial assistant: **Stephanie Camangian**
Formatting/page make-up: **TSI Graphics, Inc.**
Printer/binder: **Victor Graphics, Inc.**
Cover design: **Miguel Ortiz**
Cover photo: **Mike Gallitelli**

Printed in the United States of America

10 9 8 7 6 5 4 3 2

ISBN 0-8359-5264-9

Prentice-Hall International (UK) Limited, *London*
Prentice-Hall of Australia Pty. Limited, *Sydney*
Prentice-Hall Canada Inc., *Toronto*
Prentice-Hall Hispanoamericana, S.A., *Mexico*
Prentice-Hall of India Private Limited, *New Delhi*
Prentice-Hall of Japan, Inc., *Tokyo*
Pearson Education Asia Pte. Ltd., *Singapore*
Editoria Prentice-Hall do Brasil, *Ltda., Rio de Janero*

Contents

To the Student

As a nursing assistant in long-term care, you have the opportunity and the obligation to make a significant difference in the day-to-day lives of those you serve. Next to the residents themselves, you are the most important member of the health-care team. You not only perform nursing tasks, but often serve as family, friend, and of course, caregiver to the resident.

By learning as much as you can about your role and responsibilities, you'll discover that your job performance improves and, along with that improvement, your feelings of satisfaction increase. By giving kind, considerate, and intelligent care, you'll be able to feel good about what you're doing. Residents, family members, fellow employees, and your supervisors will recognize and respond to your good care.

The authors have endeavored to develop a learning program consisting of textbook, workbook, and instructor's guide to make learning easy and fun. To achieve the most from this program, read each lesson in the text before it is covered in class. This allows you to ask questions that arise during your reading and to contribute to class discussion. Following the class, complete the workbook assignments. If you make errors in one area, go back to the text and reread the material. Ask questions for clarification.

This training will result not only in your gaining knowledge, but also in your developing new attitudes and skills. To learn skills, practice is necessary. First, you'll observe the skill being demonstrated for you. Pay close attention. Next, you'll probably practice in class using either a classmate as a model or a mannequin. This is the time when you'll work the kinks out of the procedure. Feel free to make mistakes. Practice until it seems easy to you. Accept the feedback on your performance as designed to help you learn and improve, not as criticism.

When practicing as you care for residents, remember that the safety of the resident and of yourself is of the highest importance. If you are unsure of how to perform a skill, ask for help. Remember the phrase, "When in doubt, don't." Many students find it helpful to discuss out loud the steps to be taken in carrying out a procedure. This serves two purposes: It informs the resident of what you are going to do, and it helps you recall all the steps before you actually carry them out.

Observe others as they carry out various skills. Find out what makes them successful, and learn from their experience. Ask senior staff members or other students for feedback.

As you begin this adventure in learning, remember to enjoy yourself. A sense of humor makes coping with any situation much easier. Don't be afraid to laugh and to have fun.

CHAPTER 1

Introduction to Long-Term Care

SECTION 1 ■ The Long-Term Care Facility

Objectives

When you have completed this section, you will be able to

- ◆ Identify the four basic functions and purposes of the long-term care facility
- ◆ List the three most common reasons residents require long-term care
- ◆ Identify three sources of payment for long-term care

Key Terminology

- ◆ long-term care (LTC) facility — a nursing care center that provides specialized health-care services to the aged and chronically ill who require short-term and long-term care and rehabilitation
- ◆ activities of daily living (ADL) — activities or tasks needed for daily living, such as eating, grooming, dressing, bathing, and toileting
- ◆ developmental disability — a condition, closely related to mental retardation, in which the client is often seriously disabled
- ◆ hospice — a health-care agency that provides care to residents who have a limited life expectancy and their families
- ◆ home health-care agencies — agencies that provide services to chronically ill, disabled, or recuperating patients in the home
- ◆ adult day-care centers — places where care is provided for those who cannot or do not want to be alone during the day

Learning Activities

1. What are the four basic functions and purposes of the LTC facility?

(1) PROVIDE CARE TO RESIDENTS BASED ON IDENTIFIED NEEDS

(2) UTILIZE MULTIDISCIPLINARY HEALTH-CARE TEAM TO PLAN CARE & PROVIDE SERVICES.

(3) PREVENT ILLNESS, INJURY, OR LOSS OF FUNCTION

(4) PROMOTE RECOVERY + HEALTH THROUGH MAINTAINING EXISTING ABILITIES + RESTORING FORMER ABILITIES

2. List the three most common reasons residents require long-term care.

(1) INABILITY TO PERFORM ADL

(2) DECREASED MENTAL ABILITIES W/ VARIOUS DEMENTIAS CAUSING CONFUSION + DIFFICULT BEHAVIORS AS WELL AS MEDICAL PROBLEMS.

(3) ABSENCE OF A CAREGIVER

3. Fill in the organizational chart shown in Figure 1–1 with the names of the appropriate people in your facility.

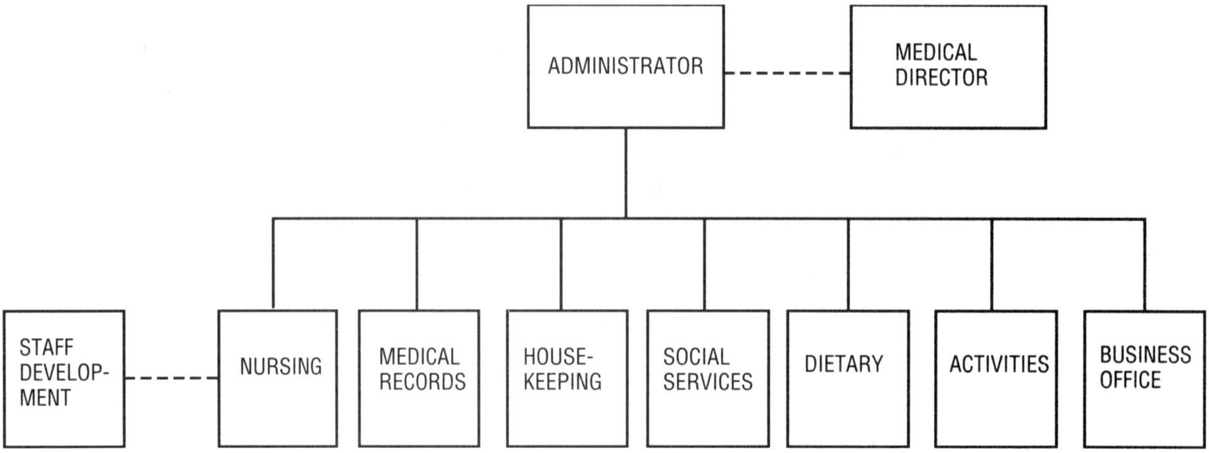

Figure 1–1
Organizational chart.

4. Identify three sources of payment for long-term care.

(1) MEDICARE

(2) MEDICADE

(3) PRIVATE

5. Identify one community resource for information regarding eligibility, services, and payment methods for long-term care.

Notes

Critical Skill Checklist for Chapter 1, Section 1

◆ Accurately complete the Learning Activities

11/6/00 Date

TJ Initial

Date of Completion 11-24-00 Instructor Carolyn Moore RN

SECTION 2 ■ The Nursing Assistant as an Employee

Objectives

When you have completed this section, you will be able to

- ◆ Define the terms *policy*, *procedure*, and *job description*
- ◆ Explain where the employer's rules for employees can be found
- ◆ Compare your job description with a sample job description

Key Terminology

- ◆ policy — describes what will be done
- ◆ procedure — describes how something is to be done
- ◆ job description — describes who will do what

Learning Activities

1. Define the terms *policy*, *procedure*, and *job description*
   a. A policy tells WHAT WILL BE DONE.
   b. A procedure describes HOW IT WILL BE DONE.
   c. A job description defines WHO IS TO DO WHAT.
2. Rules for employee behavior can be found in the facility's PERSON. POLICY HANDBOOK.
3. Draw an organizational chart for the department of nursing in your facility, using the appropriate titles and names.

4. How is your job description different from the sample included in Figure 1–2?

Figure 1-2 Sample job description.

Nursing Service:	Nursing assistant
Position Summary:	The nursing assistant is responsible for providing direct resident care under the supervision of the charge nurse. The nursing assistant follows established facility policies and procedures while providing care and coordinates resident care with other facility personnel and families.
Position Relationships	
Responsible to:	Charge nurse Treatment nurse Nurse supervisor Director of nursing
Workers Supervised:	None
Interrelationships:	Director of nursing Nurse supervisor Charge nurse Treatment nurse Other department supervisors Physicians Families Consultant personnel Ancillary service purveyors
Qualifications	
Education:	High school diploma desirable
Personal:	Presents a neat, well-groomed appearance Good physical and emotional health

Job Description

1. Follows established performance standards and performs duties according to nursing service policies and procedures.
2. Requests clarification and/or training for policies and procedures that are not clearly understood.
3. Assists new employees in following established hospital policies and procedures.
4. Provides direct resident care as assigned, completing assignments accurately and in a timely manner.
5. Identifies special resident problems and reports immediately to the charge nurse.
6. Conducts resident rounds daily and initiates corrective action immediately.
7. Identifies safety hazards and emergency situations and initiates corrective action immediately.
8. Provides nursing care to residents without violating the Resident's Bill of Rights.
9. Participates in facility education programs as assigned (i.e., orientation, in-service, and precertification) and coordinates training needs with the director of staff development.

10. Attends all classes as assigned and completes assignments accurately and on time.
11. Demonstrates an attitude of cooperation and enthusiasm in classroom and resident care activities.
12. Assumes personal responsibility for following facility procedures related to the control of equipment and supplies within the unit.
13. Assumes accountability for compliance with federal, state, and local regulations within the unit assigned and within the span of control of the nursing assistant.
14. Reports to the charge nurse or nurse supervisor any unusual problems or incidents as well as the failure of fellow employees to adhere to established policies and procedures.
15. Accurately documents incidents or unusual problems following established facility procedures.
16. Demonstrates consistent ability to work cooperatively with residents, charge nurses, treatment nurses, restorative assistants, other nursing assistants, physicians, families, consulting personnel, and ancillary service purveyors.
17. Participates in resident care conferences and other facility meetings as assigned.
18. Participates in the development of an individualized plan of resident care for residents assigned. Reviews care plan daily and performs nursing care as outlined.
19. Provides nursing care as outlined by the charge nurse and the resident care plan.
20. Documents, in the nurse assistant notes on each shift of duty, the care and treatment provided to the resident and the resident's response or lack of response to the care provided. ADL Book
21. Reports changes in resident condition immediately to the charge nurse or nurse supervisor.
22. Seeks assistance when confronted with a resident problem that requires special assessment.
23. Performs basic nursing skills as outlined in the facility education program, demonstrating knowledge and competence.
24. Follows facility procedures for admission, discharge, and transfer of residents. Completes all documentation accurately.
25. Greets residents by name and speaks to residents and family members in a kind and thoughtful manner.
26. Listens to resident and family complaints attentively and reports problems promptly to the charge nurse.
27. Responds appropriately to the feelings of others by listening attentively and taking follow-up action.
28. Controls angry feelings and only expresses anger in appropriate areas.
29. Demonstrates concern for the welfare of all residents by rendering immediate assistance to *any* resident in need.
30. Answers call lights promptly.

31. Demonstrates warm, caring feelings about residents by responding appropriately to their needs.
32. Works wherever assigned with a cooperative spirit.
33. Comes to work as scheduled and consistently demonstrates dependability.
34. Comes to work on time and consistently demonstrates punctuality.
35. Comes to work in a clean, neat uniform and consistently adheres to the dress code.

Notes

Critical Skill Checklist for Chapter 1, Section 2

◆ Accurately complete the Learning Activities   11/6/00 Date   TJ Initial

Date of Completion 11-24-00   Instructor Carolyn Moore RN

SECTION 3 ■ Legal and Ethical Responsibilities

Objectives

When you have completed this section, you will be able to

- ◆ Identify actions that are unethical or illegal
- ◆ Identify situations in which a resident's rights are being violated
- ◆ Define the terms *libel* and *slander*
- ◆ List three ways the nursing assistant can help prevent theft and loss of residents' personal property

Key Terminology

- legal — according to the laws of the community, state, or nation
- Resident Rights — a written federal regulation that defines the rights guaranteed to residents
- negligence — the failure to act as an average person would act under the same circumstances
- gross negligence — when the person responsible shows so little care that it appears that he or she is indifferent to the welfare of others
- assault — a threat or an unsuccessful attempt to commit bodily harm
- battery — an assault that is successfully carried out, injuring the victim in some way
- false imprisonment — detaining or restraining a person without proper consent
- elder abuse — physical, mental, or financial mistreatment of an elderly person
- code of ethics — a code of conduct for a particular group of people
- confidentiality — a guarantee of a resident's right to privacy
- invasion of privacy — when personal information about a resident is exposed publicly
- chart — the resident's written health record, which is a legal document
- defamation of character — making false or damaging statements about another person that injure his or her reputation
- slander — a spoken statement of defamation of character
- libel — a written statement of defamation of character

Resident Rights

The resident has a right to a dignified existence, self-determination, and communication with and access to persons and services inside and outside the facility. A facility must protect and promote the rights of each resident, including each of the following rights:

The resident has the right to exercise his or her rights as a resident of the facility and as a citizen or resident of the United States.

The resident has the right to be free of interference, coercion, discrimination, or reprisal from the facility in exercising his or her rights.

In the case of a resident adjudged incompetent under the laws of a state by a court of competent jurisdiction, the rights of the resident are exercised by the person appointed under state law to act on the resident's behalf.

The resident has the right to inspect and purchase photocopies of all records pertaining to the resident, upon written request and 48 hours' notice to the facility.

The resident has the right to be fully informed in language that he or she can understand of his or her total health status, including but not limited to his or her medical condition.

The resident has the right to refuse treatment, and to refuse to participate in experimental research.

The resident has the right to manage his or her financial affairs and the facility may not require residents to deposit their personal funds with the facility.

The resident has the right to choose a personal attending physician.

The resident has the right to be fully informed in advance about care and treatment and of treatment that may affect the resident's well-being.

The resident has the right, unless judged incompetent or otherwise found to be incapacitated under the laws of the state, to participate in planning care and treatment or changes in care and treatment.

The resident has the right to personal privacy and confidentiality of his or her personal and clinical records. Personal privacy includes accommodations, medical treatment, written and telephone communications, personal care, and visits and meetings with family and resident groups.

The resident has the right to voice grievances with respect to treatment or care that is or fails to be furnished, without discrimination or reprisal for voicing the grievances.

The resident has the right to prompt efforts by the facility to resolve grievances the resident may have, including those with respect to the behavior of other residents.

The resident has the right to examine the results of the most recent survey of the facility conducted by federal or state surveyors and any plan of correction in effect with respect to the facility.

The resident has the right to receive information from agencies acting as client advocates, and to be afforded the opportunity to contract agencies.

The resident has the right to refuse to perform services for the facility.

The resident has the right to perform services for the facility, if he or she chooses.

The resident has the right to privacy in written communications, including the right to send mail and receive promptly mail that is unopened; and to have access to stationery, postage, and writing implements at the resident's own expense.

The resident has the right to have regular access to the private use of a telephone.

The resident has the right to be free from any physical restraints imposed or psychoactive drugs administered for purposes of discipline or convenience and not required to treat the resident's medical symptoms.

Learning Activities

1. Read the following list of actions, and circle the letter of those that are considered illegal or unethical.

   a. The nursing assistant takes food from a resident's tray.
   b. The nursing assistant is unable to report to work due to a death in the family. She gives notice.
   c. The nursing assistant stays home from work to prepare for a party.
   d. The nursing assistant calls home using the telephone at the nursing station.
   e. The nursing assistant reports a co-worker for verbally abusing a resident.

2. Which of the following situations show a resident's rights being violated?

   a. Mrs. Smith cannot open her mail. At her request, a nursing assistant opens a letter and reads it to her.
   b. All outgoing mail is opened at the Business Office to be sure no false information is being sent out.
   c. A resident asks the nursing assistant to take him to the telephone. The nursing assistant refuses because she believes the resident is confused.
   d. The family is asked to take all personal items home because there is too little space in the resident's room.

3. Defamation of character that is spoken is called Slander.
   Defamation of character that is written is called liable.

4. List three ways the nursing assistant can help prevent theft and loss of residents' personal belongings.

   (1) MARK ITEMS

   (2) INVENTORY

   (3) REPORT SUSPICIOUS ACTIVITY

Notes

Critical Skill Checklist for Chapter 1, Section 3

- Accurately complete the Learning Activities — Date: 11/6/00 — Initial: TF
- Complete a resident's personal inventory form, and verify its accuracy and completeness with the instructor. — Date: ______ — Initial: ______

Date of Completion 11-24-00 Instructor Carolyn Moore, RN

SECTION 4 ■ Personal Qualities

Objectives

When you have completed this section, you will be able to

- Evaluate yourself by completing the personal qualities assessment
- Determine whether you are a good listener
- Explain how to tell the difference between information that should remain private and information that should be passed on to the charge nurse
- List the five traits that are most beneficial in a helping relationship
- Give two examples of acceptable ways to control angry feelings
- Give three examples of what it means to be dependable

Key Terminology

- communication — a method of exchanging ideas through speech, writing, or signals; requires a sender, a message, and a receiver
- touch — a form of communication that involves physical contact
- empathy — the ability to put yourself in another's place and to see things as that person sees them
- respect — recognition of the worth of another person
- genuineness — being yourself; not pretending to be different from what you are
- warmth — the demonstration of concern and affection for others
- caring — understanding the fears, problems, and distress of others, combined with a desire to help
- behaving courteously — putting the needs of others before your own
- tact — the ability to say or do the right thing at the right time

Learning Activities

1. Complete the personal qualities assessment in Figure 1-3.
2. When trying to decide what resident information should remain private and what should be reported to the charge nurse, the nursing assistant should ask these two questions:
   (1) Does the info. need to be passed on because it would have some bearing on the residents care?
   (2) Does the person to whom I'll relate this info need it in order to plan or provide care?
3. In establishing a helping relationship, these five qualities are beneficial:
   (1) Empathy
   (2) Respect
   (3) Genuinieness
   (4) Warmth
   (5) Caring
4. Emotional control is necessary when working as a nursing assistant. List two acceptable ways to express anger.
   (1) Physical activity
   (2) Talk - say, "I am angry."
5. List three ways the nursing assistant demonstrates dependability.
   (1) REPORT TO WORK ON TIME
   (2) KEEP ABSENCE TO MINIMUM
   (3) KEEP PROMISES.

Notes

Critical Skill Checklist for Chapter 1, Section 4

- Accurately complete the Learning Activities — Date: 11/6/00 — Initial: [illegible]
- Practice the use of the five traits essential to the helping relationship, and report the results to the instructor. — Date: ______ — Initial: ______

Date of Completion 11-24-00 Instructor Carolyn Moore, RN

Figure 1–3 Personal qualities assessment.

	Always	*Almost Always*	*Sometimes*	*Hardly Ever*	*Never*
A. Personal Integrity					
1. I keep confidential information to myself.	✓				
2. How I act and what I say are the same.		✓			
3. I am a caring person.	✓				
4. I am courteous and polite in my dealings with others.		✓			
5. I control my temper.	✓				
6. I tell the truth.	✓				
7. I can be depended on to do what I say I'll do.	✓				
8. I believe my work is important.	✓				
9. I am eager to learn new things.		✓			
10. I treat others with dignity and respect.	✓				
B. Interpersonal Profile					
1. I am a good listener.		✓			
2. I can express my thoughts and ideas easily.		✓			
3. I can put myself in another's place and see things as he or she sees them.		✓			
4. I am concerned about others and can express my concern in an affectionate way.	✓				
5. I can express myself tactfully.		✓			
6. I enjoy working with others.	✓				
7. I respect others even when their beliefs and opinions are different from mine.	✓				
C. Personal Health/Hygiene					
1. I bathe and shampoo regularly.	✓				
2. I am free of offensive odors.	✓				
3. I keep my hair clean and well groomed.	✓				
4. My nails are clean and are an appropriate length.	✓				
5. I eat well-balanced meals.		✓			
6. I exercise regularly.			✓		
7. I get adequate sleep.		✓			

Figure 1–3 Personal qualities assessment. (continued)

	Always	*Almost Always*	*Sometimes*	*Hardly Ever*	*Never*
D. Personal Work Habits					
1. I report to work as scheduled.		✓			
2. I report to work on time.	✓				
3. I follow the facility dress code, always wearing clean, well-fitting clothes or uniform.	✓				
4. I follow the facility's rules.	✓				
5. I do my work as assigned.	✓				
6. I plan and organize my work.		✓			
7. I volunteer to help others when I see they need help—before they ask for it.		✓			
8. I finish my work on time.		✓			
9. I seek help if I have questions.		✓			
10. I accurately document the care given and the response to that care.	✓				

I would like to work on Staying rested/well & being a little more confident.

I can start by having a better outlook, not being so "Stressed".

My progress: ______.

SECTION 5 ■ The Health-Care Team

Objectives

When you have completed this section, you will be able to

- ◆ Describe your goal for higher or continuing education and list the steps necessary to reach that goal
- ◆ Match the members of the health-care team with their major responsibilities

Key Terminology

- ◆ teamwork — work done by several people who know what is to be done and do it to the best of their ability with a spirit of cooperation
- ◆ multidisciplinary — when professional people with different educational backgrounds work together

Figure 1–4 Roles and responsibilities of the health-care team.

Health Team Member	Education	Licensing	Responsibilities
Physician, Psychiatrist For more information, write to: American Medical Association 535 N. Dearborn Chicago, IL 60610	Bachelor's degree and graduation from medical school; internship and residency required	Licensed by the state	Diagnoses medical, emotional, and social problems Orders medications, treatments, and therapy and evaluates residents' response Guides residents' plan of care and heads the health-care team
Hospital Administrator For more information, write to: American Health Care Association 1200 15th St., N.W. Washington, DC 20005	Requirements vary in each state; special educational degrees, courses, and/or experience required	Licensed by the state	Assumes total responsibility for the overall function of the long-term care facility Meets with families and community agencies to plan and provide for special resident needs Monitors the overall services provided to ensure that federal and state regulations are implemented Participates in facility educational programs
Registered Nurse (RN) For more information, write to: National League for Nursing 10 Columbus Circle New York, NY 10019 American Nurses Association 10 Columbus Circle New York, NY 10019	Three basic kinds of educational preparation: • Bachelor's degree (BSN) • Associate degree (ADN) • Three-year hospital-based nursing school diploma program	Licensed by the state	Directs and supervises all resident care and activities Plans, schedules, and assigns resident care Assesses resident problems and needs and initiates the health-care plan in coordination with other disciplines Evaluates the care provided Provides direct care—gives medications and treatments Interacts with the physician, other disciplines, residents, families, and visitors Teaches nursing principles and tasks to other nursing personnel Supervises nursing department employees
Licensed Vocational Nurse (LVN), Licensed Practical Nurse (LPN) For more information, write to: National Federation of Licensed Practical Nurses, Inc. PO Box 11038 Durham, NC 27703	One-year program	Licensed by the state	Plans, organizes, and supervises the care provided in the assigned area Provides direct nursing care—gives medications and treatments Documents the care provided and residents' response to that care Teaches nursing care skills to the nursing assistant

Figure 1–4 Roles and responsibilities of the health-care team. (continued)

Health Team Member	Education	Licensing	Responsibilities
Pharmacy Consultant For more information, write to: American Pharmaceutical Association 2215 Constitution Ave. N.W. Washington, DC 20037 National Association of Retail Druggists 1750 K St., N.W. Washington, DC 20006	Bachelor's degree (minimum); many programs offer doctorate degrees in pharmacy	Licensed by the state	Provides the facility administrator with supervisory services for developing and coordinating all pharmaceutical services Maintains regularly scheduled visits to determine that pharmacy policies and procedures are implemented correctly Reviews and documents monthly the drug regimens of each resident and recommends changes as necessary Participates in the educational development of licensed nursing personnel
Dentist For more information, write to: American Dental Association 211 E. Chicago Ave. Chicago, IL 60611	Bachelor's degree and graduation from dental school; internship and residency required	Licensed by the state	Assists the administrator in planning the facility's dental health policies and procedures Participates in facility educational programs Consults with the attending physician and recommends dental care and treatment for specific residents
Doctor of Podiatric Medicine (DPM) For more information, write to: American Podiatry Association 20 Chevy Chase, N.W. Washington, DC 20015	Bachelor's degree and graduation from podiatry school	Licensed by the state	Consults with the attending physician and recommends podiatry care and treatment of the feet for specific residents Participates in facility education programs related to the care of the feet
Medical Record Consultant For more information, write to: American Medical Records Association 875 N. Michigan Ave., Suite 1850 Chicago, IL 60611	Registered Record Administrator (RRA)—bachelor's degree Accredited Record Technician (ART)—associate arts degree	Registered or accredited by the American Medical Records Association	Provides the administrator with a plan for maintaining clinical health records and protecting medical records' information Instructs and supervises facility-employed medical records personnel Audits medical records for required entries and completeness and makes recommendations as necessary

Figure 1–4 Roles and responsibilities of the health-care team. (continued)

Health Team Member	Education	Licensing	Responsibilities
Medical Records Designee For more information, write to: American Medical Records Association 875 N. Michigan Ave., Suite 1850 Chicago, IL 60611	Requirements vary in each state (generally on-the-job training)	Some RRA or ART programs offer a certificate	Works under the direction of the medical records consultant Manages the day-to-day processing, handling, and storage of records
Occupational Therapist, Registered (OTR), Certified Occupational Therapy Assistant (OTA) For more information, write to: American Occupational Therapy Association 1383 Picard Dr. Rockville, MD 20850	Bachelor's degree	Registered by the American Occupational Therapy Association Certified by the American Occupational Therapy Association	Provides the facility administrator with a plan for occupational therapy services Assesses and documents residents' needs for occupational therapy services per physician orders and reports progress Provides therapy and recommends the use of splinting and assistive devices to help residents achieve greater levels of independence in activities of daily living associated with the upper extremities Participates in the educational development of facility staff
Speech Therapist, Audiologist For more information, write to: National Speech and Hearing Association 814 Thayer Ave., #202 Silver Spring, MD 20910	Bachelor's degree (minimum)	Licensed by the state Certified by the American Speech and Hearing Association	Provides the facility administrator with a plan for speech and hearing services Assesses and documents residents' needs for speech and hearing therapy Provides therapy under the direction of the physician and reports progress Participates in the educational development of facility staff
Recreational Therapist (May serve as activity director or consultant to the activities coordinator) For more information, write to: National Therapeutic Recreation Society 3101 Park Center Dr. Alexandria, VA 22302	Bachelor's degree	Licensed or registered by the state Registered by the National Therapeutic Recreation and Park Association	Provides the facility administrator with a plan for an activity program Assesses and documents resident's needs for recreational therapy Plans, organizes, and conducts the facility activity program or supervises the activities coordinator in doing so Participates in the educational development of facility staff

Figure 1–4 Roles and responsibilities of the health-care team. (continued)

Health Team Member	Education	Licensing	Responsibilities
Activities Coordinator	May be a recreational therapist, occupational therapist, or occupational therapy assistant or may have experience in activities in a health-care setting		Works under the direction of professional consultant Plans, organizes, and supervises activity functions Documents participation in and response to activity functions
Social Service Worker (May be employed by the facility on a full-time basis or on a part-time basis as a consultant) For more information, write to: National Association of Social Workers 1425 H St., N.W., Suite 600 Washington, DC 20005	Bachelor's degree or masters degree	Licensed by the state	Provides the facility administrator with a plan for the operation of social services according to state and federal guidelines Provides consultation for the facility-employed social service designee Assesses and documents residents' social needs and plans care to meet identified needs Participates in the educational development of facility staff
Social Service Designee	Requirements vary in each state; vocational training usually required (40-60 hours)	Most programs issue a certificate of completion	Provides services under the direction of the social service consultant Assists residents and family with arrangements for admission, discharge, and transfer Assesses, evaluates, and documents residents' social needs and financial needs
Respiratory Therapist For more information, write to: National Board of Respiratory Care 8310 Nieman Rd. Lenexa, KS 66214	Bachelor's degree	Licensed by the state	Provides the facility administrator with a plan for the operation of respiratory therapy services Assesses and documents residents' needs for respiratory therapy services per physician's orders and reports progress
Registered Physical Therapist (RPT) (May be employed by the facility on a full-time basis or on a part-time basis as a consultant) For more information, write to: American Physical Therapy Association 1156 15th St., N.W. Washington, DC 20005	Bachelor's degree	Licensed by the state or registered by the American Registry of Physical Therapists	Provides the facility administrator with a plan for the operation of physical therapy services according to state and federal guidelines Assesses and documents residents' needs for physical therapy per physician's orders and reports progress Assists residents to improve their mobility through ambulation, gait training, and transfer techniques

Figure 1–4 Roles and responsibilities of the health-care team. (continued)

Health Team Member	Education	Licensing	Responsibilities
			Participates in the educational development of facility staff
Registered Dietitian (RD) (May be employed by the facility on a full-time basis or on a part-time basis as a consultant) For more information, write to: American Dietetic Association 430 North Michigan Ave. Chicago, IL 60611	Bachelor's degree and one-year internship	Licensed by the American Dietetic Association	Provides the facility administrator with a plan for the operation of dietary services according to state and federal regulations Plans, prepares, and evaluates menu Contributes to the health-care plan Participates in the educational development of facility staff Assesses and documents residents' nutritional needs and recommends changes to physicians and nursing staff
Dietary Service Supervisor (DSS)	Special vocational training (average 40-60 hours) usually required	Some programs issue a certificate of completion	Works under the direction of the dietitian Plans, organizes, and schedules dietary services and orders, stores, prepares, and serves food

Learning Activities

1. Review Figure 1-4, and take time to consider your career goals. What do you want to be doing five years from now? On a separate sheet of paper, write down your goals, then make a "Things to Do" list of the steps you need to take to reach your goals. These may include contacting some of the organizations listed in the figure or enrolling in a class. Cross out each step as you accomplish it. Add to the list as you learn more.

2. Match the health-care team members in column A with the major responsibilities in column B.

Column A

F physical therapist

E occupational therapist

A registered nurse

D licensed practical/ vocational nurse

C nursing assistant

B physician

Column B

a. identifies resident problems and supervises the implementation of the plan of care

b. leads the health-care team

c. provides direct care to residents, under the direction of a licensed nurse, according to the approved plan of care

d. administers medications and treatments

e. is concerned primarily with upper extremity function, as in feeding, dressing, and grooming

f. works primarily with lower extremity functions, as in transferring and ambulation

Notes

Critical Skill Checklist for Chapter 1, Section 5

◆ Accurately complete the Learning Activities.	11/6/00 Date	TJ Initial
◆ Write for information regarding your special field of interest.	Date	Initial
◆ Identify the members of the health-care team in your LTC facility by name and title.	Date	Initial

Date of Completion 11-24-00 Instructor Carolyn Moore, RN

CHAPTER 2

Your Working Environment

SECTION 1 ■ Emergencies and Accident Prevention

Objectives

When you have completed this section, you will be able to

- Give four examples of the ways the nursing assistant helps to prevent residents from falling
- Select three ways the nursing assistant can help prevent residents being burned
- Demonstrate the application of a soft protective device
- Identify situations in which protective devices may be used
- Define *gravity*, *base of support*, and *center of gravity*
- Recognize safety hazards
- Demonstrate how to lift an object using proper body mechanics

Key Terminology

- gatch — a bed adjustment handle
- postural support — a soft protective device
- restraint — a device designed to hold back or limit a resident's movements
- body mechanics — a special way of standing and moving your body to avoid back strain and injury
- gravity — the attraction of the earth for an object on or near its surface
- center of gravity — area where the mass or bulk of an object is concentrated
- base of support — the base or foundation of an object or person

Learning Activities

1. List four ways the nursing assistant can help prevent resident falls.

   (1) Answer Call light promptly

   (2) Potion Pt. properly in bed, wheel chairs, etc

   (3) Set brakes on Chairs, beds, Commodes, etc

   (4) Bed "gatch" should be "in" (position)

2. Which three of the following can prevent burns?

   (a.) Following smoking regulations
   b. Giving residents only cold liquids
   (c.) Protecting residents from overexposure to sunlight
   (d.) Following instructions for the use of heat lamps and heating pads

3. For each of the following situations, indicate with *yes* or *no* whether soft protective devices may be applied.

   __Y__ a. Mr. Jones keeps trying to climb out of bed to go to the bathroom. He needs help because he's unsteady on his feet. The doctor's order says "soft restraints PRN safety."

   __N__ b. Mrs. Brown was spitting and cursing at the staff. She is placed in her bed with a restraint until she apologizes. There is a doctor's order that says "soft restraints PRN safety."

   __N__ c. Mrs. Green keeps wheeling her wheelchair into the nurses' station. The nursing assistant ties the wheelchair to the handrail.

   __Y__ d. The nurse is going to insert a catheter into a resident's bladder. The resident keeps trying to push her away. The nurse restrains both hands until the catheter is inserted.

4. Match the terms in column A with the definitions in column B.

Column A	Column B
__C__ gravity	a. the base or foundation of an object or person
__A__ base of support	b. the place where the bulk of an object is concentrated
__B__ center of gravity	c. the attraction of the earth for an object on or near its surface

5. Tour your facility, and identify and report any of the following safety hazards.

   ______ Spills on the floor
   ______ Objects or obstacles on the floor
   ______ Loose or broken handrails
   ______ Bed gatches out
   ______ Harmful substances accessible to residents
   ______ Call cords not within reach of residents
   ______ Residents improperly positioned in wheelchairs
   ______ Smoking in nondesignated areas
   ______ Other

6. Complete the safety crossword puzzle shown in Figure 2-1.

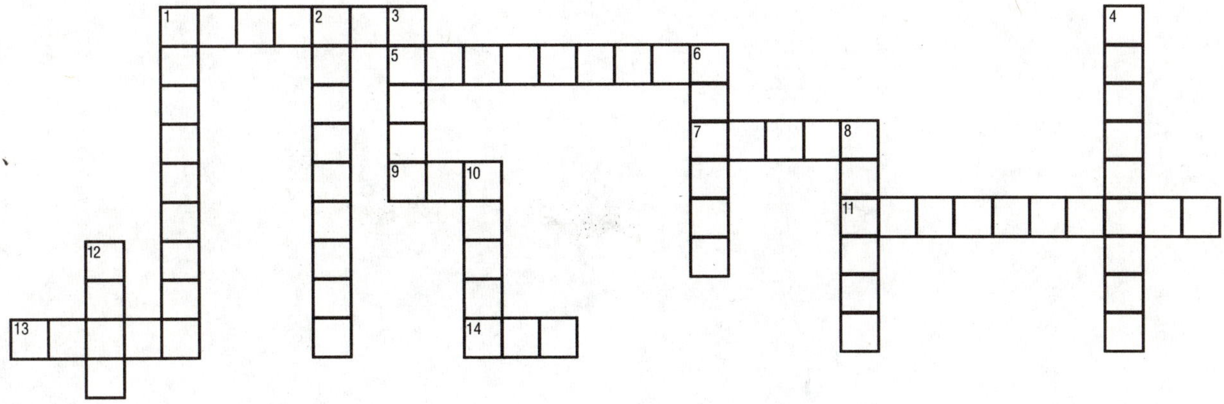

Figure 2–1
Safety crossword puzzle.

ACROSS

1. Smoking must be done in designated areas only.
5. Falls, strains, burns, and punctures are all types of Accidents.
7. The most common type of resident accident is Falls.
9. Hot liquids are a common cause of burns.
11. Restraints of any type should only be used to protect the resident from injury to self or others.
13. The second most common hazard to residents is Burns.
14. Soft Tie restraints should never restrict circulation.

DOWN

1. Siderails must be up and locked in position for all residents at night unless the charge nurse instructs you differently.
2. You must report any incident that lead you to believe that a resident is a danger to self or others.
3. The handle for the bed adjustment is often called the bed Gatch.
4. Good body Mechanics are necessary to prevent injury to yourself and others.
6. You must always protect the welfare and Safety of each resident.
8. A common type of back injury is called a Strain.
10. When providing care, avoid movements that Twist your body.
12. It takes three things to start a Fire.

Notes

Critical Skill Checklist for Chapter 2, Section 1

◆ Accurately complete the Learning Activities.	11/7/00 Date	Initial
◆ Demonstrate applying a soft protective device.	11/7/00 Date	Initial
◆ Demonstrate lifting an object using proper body mechanics.	11/7/00 Date	Initial

Date of Completion 11-24-00 Instructor Carolyn Moore, RN

Section 2 ■ Fire Safety and Disaster Preparedness

Objectives

When you have completed this section, you will be able to

- ◆ List the three things necessary to start a fire
- ◆ Identify four major causes of fires in LTC facilities
- ◆ Complete a fire prevention inspection checklist for your facility
- ◆ Describe the correct sequence of steps to be taken in the event of a fire
- ◆ Explain why the nursing assistant must know disaster plans before a disaster occurs

Key Terminology

- ◆ spontaneous combustion — the ignition of burnable materials, caused by a chemical reaction
- ◆ disaster — some type of catastrophe

Learning Activities

1. What three things are necessary to start a fire?

   (1) Heat

   (2) Fuel

   (3) Oxygen

2. List four major causes of fires in LTC facilities.

   (1) Smoking/Matches

   (2) Defects in heating systems

   (3) Improper trash disposal

   (4) Spontanious ignition

3. Complete the fire prevention inspection checklist in Figure 2-2 for your LTC facility

4. For the following situation, describe the correct sequence of steps to be taken. Nursing assistant Mary Jane is walking down the hallway when she smells smoke. She searches for the origin, then notices smoke coming from the open doorway of Room 101. Upon entering the room, she finds that the trash can and bedside cabinet are on fire. Mrs. Smith, a dependent resident, is lying in the bed yelling for help.

   (1) Rescue

   (2) Alert/Report

   (3) Confine

   (4) Extinguish

5. Why must a nursing assistant know disaster plans before a disaster occurs? To quickly evacuate/act if + when something happens. Remove pt./records, etc.

Critical Skill Checklist for Chapter 2, Section 2

◆ Accurately complete the Learning Activities.

Date 11/7/00 Initial 7J

Date of Completion 11-24-00 Instructor Carolyn Moore, RN

Figure 2–2 Fire prevention inspection checklist.

For any problems identified, list the area, room number, resident's name, etc., so that corrective action can be taken.

SMOKING

1. List the designated smoking areas in your facility

2. Are there large noncombustible ashtrays in these areas?	yes ______	no ______
3. Is anyone smoking in nonsmoking areas?	yes ______	no ______
4. Is anyone smoking in bed without the supervision of a facility employee?	yes ______	no ______
5. Are smoking materials, such as matches and cigarette lighters, visible?	yes ______	no ______

ELECTRICAL EQUIPMENT AND HEATING

1. Are electrical cords in good condition?	yes ______	no ______
2. Are outlets in good condition?	yes ______	no ______
3. Do all plugs have three prongs?	yes ______	no ______
4. Are vents and flues clean?	yes ______	no ______

SPONTANEOUS COMBUSTION

1. Is there any area that appears to have a lot of litter?	yes ______	no ______
2. Are rubbish and trash areas clean and litter-free?	yes ______	no ______

USE OF OXYGEN

1. Is a "No-Smoking" sign posted when oxygen is in use?	yes ______	no ______
2. Are there any flammable materials, such as matches and lighters, stored in a room where oxygen is being used?	yes ______	no ______
3. Are stored oxygen cylinders chained or strapped securely to a wall, stand, or cart?	yes ______	no ______

OTHER

1. Is there any evidence of flammable liquids that have not been properly stored?	yes ______	no ______
2. Are fire exits properly lighted?	yes ______	no ______
3. Are fire exits free from clutter and obstacles?	yes ______	no ______

4. List the locations of the fire extinguishers in your assigned work area.

5. List the locations of the fire alarms in your assigned work area.

SECTION 3 ■ Infection Control

Objectives

When you complete this section, you will be able to

- Define the terms *organism, microorganism, pathogenic, nonpathogenic,* and *aseptic*
- List ways that microorganisms are spread
- List four signs of infection
- Define the terms *isolation, disinfection,* and *sterilization*
- Identify areas that are considered clean and those that are considered dirty
- Give two examples of materials that are considered infectious waste
- Demonstrate proper hand-washing technique
- Demonstrate proper linen-handling procedures
- Explain when standard precautions are to be used
- List the three types of precautions that are used in addition to standard precautions
- Explain when gloves should be worn

Key Terminology

- organism — any living thing
- microorganism (commonly called *germs*) — tiny living things seen only with a microscope
- pathogenic — causing disease
- nonpathogenic — not capable of producing disease
- infection — the invasion of the body by a disease-producing organism
- aseptic — free of microorganisms
- incidence — the number of occurrences
- culture — a sample of infected material that is sent to a laboratory to be studied
- feces — solid human waste
- toxins — waste products of microorganisms that act like poison in the body
- cross-infection — an infection that residents, employees, families, or visitors acquire from someone else
- reinfection — a second occurrence of an infection in one individual
- exposure — coming into contact with a microorganism without the tissues being invaded
- environmental control — maintaining an environment as free as possible of pathogenic organisms
- isolation — separating or setting apart

- disinfection — the process of using a chemical substance to kill most microorganisms
- sterilization — the process of using several different methods to kill all microorganisms
- autoclaving — a method of sterilization that uses pressurized steam at a high temperature
- sterile — free from all microorganisms
- contaminated — not sterile
- clean — uncontaminated or free from pathogenic organisms, but not sterile
- dirty — contaminated, used, or exposed to people or places where disease-producing organisms are present
- infectious — having come in contact with a person with an infection or communicable disease that could be carried or transmitted
- infectious waste — any disposable item that contains body discharges (e.g., saliva, wound drainage, urine, feces)
- standard precautions — guidelines developed to protect health-care workers, residents, and visitors from the spread of infectious diseases

---

Learning Activities

1. Match the terms in column A with the definitions in column B.

Column A	Column B
__D__ microorganism	a. causing disease
__C__ organism	b. not capable of producing disease
__A__ pathogenic	c. any living thing
__B__ nonpathogenic	d. tiny living things seen only with a microscope
__E__ aseptic	e. free of microorganisms

2. How can microorganisms be spread? Circle the correct answers.
   - (a.) Touching the resident
   - (b.) Touching the bed linens
   - (c.) Sneezing
   - (d.) Contaminated food or water
   - (e.) Dust in the air

3. List four signs of infection that should be noted and reported.

   (1) Fever

   (2) Pain

   (3) Redness

   (4) Draining fluids ~ eyes, nose, ears.

4. Explain what is meant by each of the following:

   a. Isolation - Separate\Set apart

   b. Disinfection - Killing Microorganisms w\Chemicals

   c. Sterilization - Killing microorganisms Steam | high temps - "autoclaving"

5. From the list below, circle the items that are considered infectious waste.

   a. Resident clothing
   b. Soiled dressings
   c. Needles and syringes
   d. Contaminated food or water
   e. Facial tissues when the resident is in isolation

6. In Figure 2–3, write next to each letter whether the item pictured is considered *clean* or *dirty*.

Figure 2–2
Resident unit.

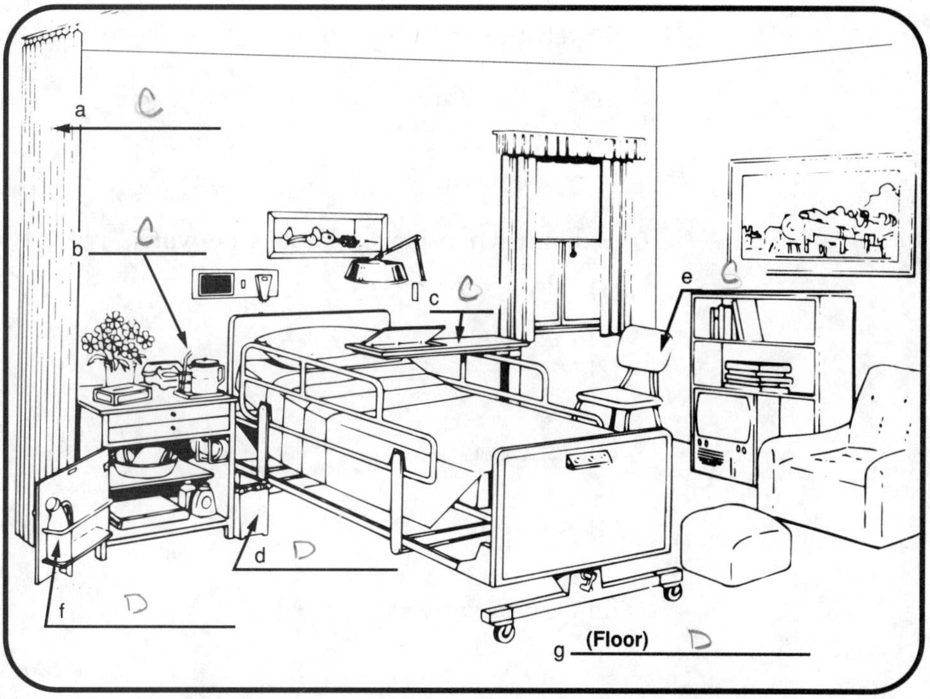

7. Mark the following statements about linen handling with a *C* if the statement is correct or with an *I* if the statement is incorrect.

C Clean linens should be stored in clean-linen areas.

I Soiled linens may be placed on the floor because both are "dirty."

C Linens taken into a resident's room may not be returned to clean-linen storage.

C Linens should not be shaken or fluffed.

I Linens dropped on the floor may be used if picked up within ten seconds.

8. Explain when standard precautions are to be used.

Mainly for blood, body fluids, excretions except sweat, whether or not they contain visible blood.

Use all the time

9. List the three types of precautions that are used in addition to standard precautions.

(1) Contact Precautions

(2) Droplet Precautions

(3) Airborne Precautions

10. Explain when gloves should be worn. Contact w/

(1) Blood

(2) Body fluids

(3) Secretions

(4) Excretions

(5) Contaminated items

Notes

Critical Skill Checklist for Chapter 2, Section 3

◆ Accurately complete the Learning Activities.	11/7/00 Date	TJ Initial
◆ Demonstrate hand-washing procedures.	11/8/00 Date	TJ Initial
◆ Demonstrate linen-handling procedures.	11/8/00 Date	Initial

Date of Completion 11-24-00 Instructor Carolyn Moore, RN

Section 4 ▪ The Resident in Isolation

Objectives

When you have completed this section, you will be able to

- ◆ Apply a mask and gown
- ◆ Describe how the nursing assistant can determine which type of isolation technique is required for a given resident
- ◆ List three ways AIDS is spread
- ◆ Describe how the nursing assistant can most effectively prevent the spread of communicable disease, including AIDS

Key Terminology

- ◆ communicable condition — the condition of someone who has an infection or disease that can be spread from one person to another
- ◆ isolation technique — any of several safety measures that separate residents from one another and require special handling of objects that have been in contact with the infected resident
- ◆ acquired immune deficiency syndrome (AIDS) —a condition in which the body's immune system is damaged by attack from a virus
- ◆ opportunistic infections — infections that occur as a result of a diseased immune system
- ◆ jaundice — a yellow coloring of the skin and the white portion of the eye, resulting from a disease process

Learning Activities

1. Describe how the nursing assistant can determine which type of isolation technique is required for a given resident.

Check for any "Signs posted." This may give the type of isolations.
Check w/ Charge nurse or any person info. from other staff.

2. List three ways AIDS is spread.

(1) Mother to Child (birth)

(2) Sexual Contact

(3) Shared needles

3. How can the nursing assistant most effectively prevent the spread of communicable disease, including AIDS?

Take strictest precautions. Wear gloves
When cleaning blood/fluids - wear gloves & use Chemicals which will kill the Virus.

Mostly — good handwashing

Notes

Critical Skill Checklist for Chapter 2, Section 4

◆ Accurately complete the Learning Activities.	11/7/00 Date	TJ Initial
◆ Demonstrate applying a mask and gown.	11/7/00 Date	TJ Initial
◆ Review any required documentation the nursing assistant must complete for a resident in isolation.	11/7/00 Date	TJ Initial

Date of Completion 11-24-00 Instructor Carolyn Moore, RN

SECTION 5 ■ The Resident's Unit: Admission and Discharge

Objectives

When you have completed this section, you will be able to

- ◆ List two ways the nursing assistant can help make the resident's unit more homelike
- ◆ Compile a list of items you would want to have with you if you were admitted to a long-term care facility
- ◆ Operate a bed and side rails
- ◆ Make an occupied bed
- ◆ Participate in a simulated admission procedure
- ◆ List four tasks to be accomplished when relocating a resident in a facility

Key Terminology

- ◆ occupied bed — a bed in which the resident remains
- ◆ unoccupied bed — a bed that the resident has left
- ◆ incontinent — lacking control over bowel and/or bladder function
- ◆ prosthesis — an artificial replacement for limbs, eyes, etc.
- ◆ transfer — to move from one place to another
- ◆ discharge — to move a resident out of the LTC facility for a long period of time or permanently

Learning Activities

1. List two ways the nursing assistant can help make the resident's unit more home-like.

   (1) Make the room ready & things accessable.

   (2) Keep the room tidy.

2. Compile a list of items you would want to have with you if you were admitted to a long-term care facility.

   Phone numbers
   Personal hygene items
   Some items from home - Pics, TV, Radio
   etc.

3. With your fellow students, act out, or role-play, admitting a resident. Use one person as the resident, one as the nursing assistant, and one as a family member. Have others take notes on how they would do it differently. Discuss afterward how each person felt.

4. When relocating a resident within a LTC facility, the nursing assistant should __inform__ the resident, give a __Careful review (Tour)__ of the new room, __introduce (orient)__ the resident to the new surroundings, and carefully gather all of the resident's __belongings__.

Notes

Critical Skill Checklist for Chapter 2, Section 5

◆ Accurately complete the Learning Activities.	11/7/00 Date	TJ Initial
◆ Review the admission, transfer, and discharge procedures for your LTC facility.	Date	Initial
◆ Accurately complete the required documentation for a new admission, a resident transfer, and a resident discharge.	Date	Initial
◆ Demonstrate operating a bed and using side rails.	✓ Date	Initial
◆ Demonstrate making an occupied bed.	✓ Date	Initial

Date of Completion 11-24-00 Instructor Carolyn Moore, RN

CHAPTER 3

Special Needs of the Elderly and Chronically Ill

SECTION 1 ■ Philosophy of Care and Rehabilitation

Objectives

When you have completed this section, you will be able to

- Give three examples of ways the nursing assistant can encourage residents to be more independent
- List three observations you have made that reflect your LTC facility's philosophy of care

Key Terminology

- philosophy — the general beliefs, concepts, and attitudes of an individual or group
- rehabilitation — restorative care in which efforts are directed to help each resident become as independent as possible
- contracture — the shortening of body muscle from inactivity
- activities of daily living (ADL) — all of the tasks and skills normally needed for daily living, such as communication, eating, grooming, dressing, bathing, walking, and toileting

Learning Activities

1. List three ways the nursing assistant can encourage residents toward greater independence.

   (1) Praise the resident for their attempts.

   (2) Overlook their failure

   (3) Allow them time to do for themselves

2. List three observations you have made that reflect your LTC facility's philosophy of care.

   (1) Compassion

   (2) Encouragement

   (3) Patience

Notes

Critical Skill Checklist for Chapter 3, Section 1

- Accurately complete the Learning Activities — 11/8/00 Date — Initial

- Interview a licensed nurse, an alert resident, and a family member, and ask them to describe their own philosophy of care. — Date — Initial

Date of Completion 11-24-00 Instructor Carolyn Moore, RN

SECTION 2 ■ Psychosocial Aspects of Aging

Objectives

When you have completed this section, you will be able to

- Define the term *psychosocial*
- List the five basic human needs that Maslow described
- Describe two ways the nursing assistant can help meet residents' need for approval and acceptance, recognition and respect, and self-esteem
- List the three developmental tasks of aging
- Complete a questionnaire about aging

Key Terminology

- psychosocial — *psycho* refers to mental or emotional processes, and *social* refers to interactions and relationships with others
- physical needs — needs that are essential to survival, such as food, water, oxygen, rest, exercise, and sex

- security needs — needs that are concerned with physical safety, feeling protected, having a job, and shelter
- social needs — the need for approval and acceptance from others
- status needs — the need for recognition and respect from others
- self-fulfillment needs — the need to achieve as fully as possible one's highest potential

---

Learning Activities

1. Define the term *psychosocial.*

   Mental/emotional process & interactions & relationships w/ others.

2. List the five basic human needs described by Maslow.

   (1) Physical (food, water, etc)

   (2) Security (safety, comfort)

   (3) Social (approval/acceptance

   (4) Status (recognition & respect)

   (5) Self fulfillment (purpose for life, participation in activities, etc).

* 3. Describe two ways the nursing assistant can help meet residents' need for each of the following.

   a. Approval and acceptance

   (1) Helping/encouragement w/ tasks

   (2) Allowing for their independence

   b. Recognition and respect

   (1) Be a good listener. Pay attention to them

   (2) Addressing them properly.

c. Self-esteem

(1) Praising | encouragement

(2) Encourage there involvement in activities.

4. Complete the questionnaire, "What Do You Know about Aging?," in Figure 3–1.

5. List the three developmental tasks of aging.

(1) Adjusting to aging, physical change

(2) Putting life (success/failure) into perspective (meaning to life)

(3) Accepting the past & focusing on the present.

Notes

Critical Skill Checklist for Chapter 3, Section 2

◆ Accurately complete the Learning Activities

11/8/00 Date

[initials] Initial

Date of Completion 11-24-00

Instructor Carolyn Moore, RN

Figure 3–1 What do you know about aging?

This is not a test. If you believe the statement is mostly correct, write *C* in the space provided. If you believe the statement is mostly incorrect, write *I* in the space provided.

__C__ 1. The aged are a rapidly growing minority.
__I__ 2. There are twice as many men in the 65-or-older age bracket than there are women.
__I__ 3. Twenty percent of the elderly live in long-term care facilities in the United States.
__C__ 4. As people age and experience some of the losses involved, friends, family, homes, and personal possessions generally become more important.
__I__ 5. The aged are always "set in their ways."
__I__ 6. Most older people are difficult to deal with and are grouchy and stubborn.
__I__ 7. People over 65 cannot learn new skills.
__I__ 8. People over 65 resent physical contact with other people.
__I__ 9. Very few people past the age of 65 are able to enjoy sexual contacts.
__I__ 10. It's usually a mistake for people over age 65 to marry.
__I__ 11. The elderly need to be taught that they will have to depend on others.
__I__ 12. Nothing can be done for the older person once confusion sets in.

Answers:

1. Correct. Since 1900, the over-65 population has grown faster than any other minority group. One in ten Americans is 65 or older. Each day, approximately 4,000 people turn 65 and about 3,000 elderly people die.
2. Incorrect. There are approximately 140 women to every 100 men in this age bracket. Most of the men are married, and most of the woman are widowed.
3. Incorrect. Approximately 4 to 5 percent of the elderly live in long-term care facilities in the United States.
4. Correct. The loss of family, friends, and homes does increase the resident's need to be surrounded by familiar things. This is why, when residents are hospitalized, they should be allowed to retain as many personal possessions as possible.
5. Incorrect. Most people are set in their ways. Generally, people who have many social contacts and varied life experiences are more flexible. However, as people grow older, social contacts frequently decrease and habits and patterns are often established, leading many people to believe that *all* flexibility is lost.
6. Incorrect. Again, personality must be considered. There are people of all ages who can be thought of as difficult or stubborn. Consider also that the hospitalized elderly are generally sick or disabled and that most people who are sick or disabled are not at their best. How do you behave and react when you are sick, depressed, or frustrated?
7. Incorrect. The elderly can and are learning new things all the time. It may take older people longer to learn a new skill or new information, but they will often retain information longer.
8. Incorrect. Many of the hospitalized elderly are isolated from the normal daily physical contacts of family and friends, and they need physical contact.
9. Incorrect. Many people are sexually active past the age of 65. It is important not to deny residents their right to sexual fulfillment.
10. Incorrect. People of *all* age need to love and be loved.
11. Incorrect. We all need to feel that we have some control over our lives. When we encourage dependence, we take away the individual's control.
12. Incorrect. Many physiological and psychological causes of confusion are treatable, and there are many nursing measures that can help residents minimize confusion.

SECTION 3 ■ Role Changes

Objectives

When you have completed this section, you will be able to

- Define the term *role*
- List the roles you play
- Differentiate the characteristics of the sick role from those of the well role
- Give three ways the nursing assistant can minimize the frustrations that accompany role changes that residents experience

Key Terminology

- role — the part a person plays in relationships with others
- well role — a role characterized by independence, responsibility, usefulness, and decision-making capability
- sick role — a role characterized by dependence, weakness, control by others, lack of responsibility, and uselessness
- disabled — being incapacitated and afflicted; neither sick nor well, but having varying degrees of both
- age appropriate — appropriate to a person's chronological age
- spiritual need — the need to find meaning in life

Learning Activities

1. Define the term *role*.

The part one plays in relationship to others.

2. Describe the roles you play in your life.

Dealing w/ those in my home
" " at work, both employees & residents
" " who are friends & loved ones.
Etc.

3. Next to each of the following characteristics, place an *S* if it is part of the sick role and a *W* if it is part of the well role.

S	Less valuable	W	Valuable
W	Independent	W	Strong
S	Dependent	W	Controlling
S	Weak	S	Controlled
W	Useful	S	Less useful

4. The nursing assistant can minimize the frustrations that accompany role changes that the residents experience by

(1) Accepting the resident & focus on how they are like us, not just on how they are different.

(2) Show interest & listen & giving full attention to them.

(3) Complying to their request when possible.

Notes

Critical Skills Checklist for Chapter 3, Section 3

◆ Accurately complete the Learning Activities 11/8/00 Date TJ Initial

Date of Completion 11-24-00 Instructor Carolyn Moore, RN

SECTION 4 ■ Developing Interpersonal Skills

Objectives

When you have completed this section, you will be able to

- List four factors influencing individual behavior
- Identify the methods of coping with anger that are acceptable for the nursing assistant
- Select the most helpful response by the nursing assistant in sample situations

Key Terminology

- heredity — the traits a person is born with
- environment — a person's surroundings, both physical and social
- culture — the habits and customs of a group
- interests — what a person enjoys or cares about
- feelings or emotions — happiness, grief, anger, jealousy, love
- values — what a person considers to be most important
- standards — what is acceptable and what is not

Learning Activities

1. List four of the factors that cause us to behave as we do.

   (1) Culture

   (2) Environment

   (3) Standards

   (4) Heredity

2. Circle the methods of coping with anger that are acceptable in a health-care setting.

   a. Slam the door and leave the room.
   b. State, "I really feel angry!"
   c. Kick the wheelchair.
   d. Discuss your feelings with the charge nurse.
   e. On your break, take a walk around the facility.
   f. Let residents and other staff know why you arc upset.
   g. Clock out and leave.

3. Circle the most helpful response in each of the following situations.

You enter James Green's room and discover him with his head in his hands, sobbing. You should

a. Slip out of the room quietly before he sees you.
b. Sit by him, take his hand, and wait for him to respond.
c. Put your arms around him and say, "Now, Mr. Green, it can't be all that bad!"
d. Ask the charge nurse if she can get the physician to order a medication to lift Mr. Green's spirits.

You enter Elizabeth Brown's room just in time to duck a water pitcher that she's hurled toward the door. You should

a. Get help so you can hold Mrs. Brown down because she's out of control.
b. Say, "Mrs. Brown, I haven't done anything to deserve that. Why did you throw the pitcher at me?"
c. Insist that Mrs. Brown apologize for her nasty temper.
d. Quietly pick up the pitcher and say, "Would you like to tell me what's happening with you? Maybe I can help."

Bill Smith has been a quadriplegic for sixteen years. You've been taking care of him for three months. Every day he describes to you in step-by-step detail how to transfer him to the wheelchair. You find yourself becoming frustrated with his continuous instruction. You should

a. Recognize his need for some control; relax, and do things as he wishes.
b. Tell him, "Mr. Smith, I know how to do it. I've been doing this every day for three months."
c. Tell him, "Look, I'm in charge here. I'm going to do it the way I want to."
d. Ask to change assignments.

Mary Jones rings her call signal every fifteen minutes. She rarely needs anything important. You should

a. Say, "Mrs. Jones, I have seven other residents to care for, some sicker than you. Please give me a break!"
b. Take the call cord away so she can't reach it.
c. Recognize the reason for her frequent calls, and ask for the help of the other members of the health-care team to try to find an approach to changing her demanding behavior.
d. Ignore the light so she thinks that it doesn't work.

Notes

Critical Skill Checklist for Chapter 3, Section 4

- Accurately complete the Learning Activities.

11/8/00 Date | Initial

- Select a resident whose behavior is often aggressive or demanding, and review the plan of care to determine whether the problem has been identified and whether approaches are being carried out consistently. Discuss these issues with the charge nurse.

Date | Initial

Date of Completion 11-24-00 Instructor Carolyn Moore RN

SECTION 5 ■ Spiritual Needs

Objectives

When you have completed this section, you will be able to

- Define the term *spiritual need*
- Choose a religious organization and describe its beliefs regarding illness and death
- Identify the activities that are appropriate to the nursing assistant's role

Key Terminology

- Spiritual need — the need to find meaning in life

Learning Activities

1. What is spiritual need?

The need to find meaning in life.

2. Choose a religious organization, and briefly describe the beliefs of the group about these topics:

a. Illness A fact of nature but strength can be gained from this experience + shared w/ others. God is w/ us even in these times.

b. Death

This is not the end. It is stepping over into another dimension of "life as an eternal spirit."

3. Review the following list of activities, and indicate with an *X* those that are appropriate to the nursing assistant's role.

_______ Invite a resident to attend church services with you.

___X___ Assist a resident to get dressed for church services at the resident's request.

_______ Comfort a dying resident by explaining that there is an afterlife.

___X___ Notify the Dietary Department that a resident does not drink coffee or tea for religious reasons.

_______ Pack up a resident's statues and pictures of Jesus, and place them in storage to eliminate clutter.

___X___ Notify the charge nurse that a resident would like to see a priest.

Notes

Critical Skill Checklist for Chapter 3, Section 5

- Accurately complete the Learning Activities.

11/8/00 Date   TJ Initial

Date of Completion 11-24-00   Instructor Carolyn Moore RN

SECTION 6 ■ The Dying Resident

Objectives

When you have completed this section, you will be able to

- Identify the goals of hospice care
- Identify the emotions that are present in each phase of the grieving process
- Participate in a simulation of a grief experience
- List two books that would help you better understand the needs of people who are dying
- Answer questions regarding policies on the care of the dying in your facility

Key Terminology

- hospice — a special kind of program that provides care for the terminally ill and their families or loved ones
- terminal illness — the last stage of an illness in which the person has a life expectancy or prognosis of six months or less
- bereave — to be left desolate by death
- grief process — the series of many different emotions experienced by people following a loss

Learning Activities

1. Identify the four goals of hospice care.

(1) To help dying person remain as free of pain as possible

(2) to allow dying person & loved ones as much control as possible

(3) To provide the highest quality of life possible when a person's time for life is limited.

(4) To assist family & loved ones after the death through bereavement counseling

2. In Figure 3–2, insert the appropriate emotions that are present in each phase of the grief process.

Figure 3–2
Stages of grief.

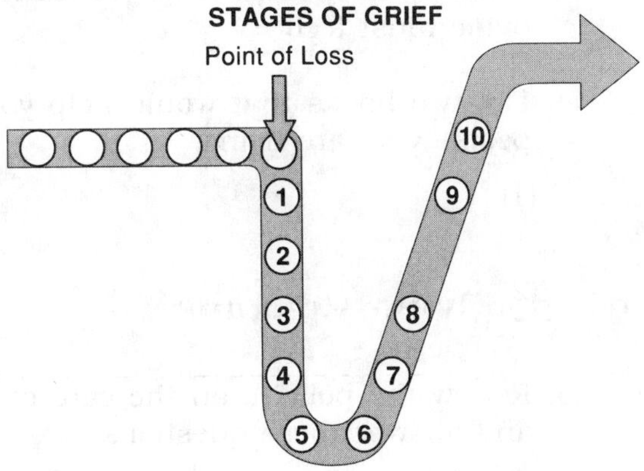

1. Frozen feelings
2. Emotional release
3. Loneliness
4. Physical symptoms
5. Guilt
6. Panic
7. Hostility
8. Selective memory
9. Struggle for new pattern
10. Life is ok.

3. In the space below, list the ten things you value most in life. These may be people, objects, or qualities, such as intelligence or health.

(1) God

(2) Special love/person

(3) Family (living + dead) memories

(4) my pets

(5) my well being/health

(6) My home

(7) Finances

(8) Future Security

(9) My special possessions

(10) Past accomplishments.

Draw a line through three of the items. Now cross off three more, and then three more. There should be only one left. Think about what it felt like. Did you experience denial (this is only paper; it doesn't count) or anger (I'm not crossing off my family!)? People who are dying lose everyone they know and everything they possess. Perhaps, in a small way, you can begin to understand the grief the dying must feel.

4. List two books that would help you better understand the needs of people who are dying. Sugg → - How TO SURVIVE the Loss of Loe - Colgro

   (1) Scripture

   (2) Real stories & those who have had their experience documented

5. Review the policies on the care of the dying in your LTC facility, and answer these questions:

   a. Are families allowed unlimited visiting?
   b. Do the clergy play a prominent role?
   c. Are residents sent to an acute-care hospital when death is imminent?
   d. What does care of the body consist of?
   e. How does the facility acknowledge the death?

Notes

Critical Skills Checklist for Chapter 3, Section 6

◆ Accurately complete the Learning Activities.

11/8/00
Date

[illegible]
Initial

Date of Completion 11-24-00

Instructor Carolyn Moore RN

CHAPTER 4

Basic Nursing Care

SECTION 1 ■ The Health-Care Plan

Objectives

When you have completed this section, you will be able to

- ◆ Review the health-care plan of ten residents in your facility and list the different health-care disciplines involved
- ◆ Explain how the nursing assistant can contribute to the development of the plan of care
- ◆ List four ways the health-care plan can help the nursing assistant provide daily care

Key Terminology

- ◆ health-care plan (often referred to as the *plan of care*) — a mini-sketch that details in writing the resident's problems, needs, and goals
- ◆ individualized — tailor-made to reflect the unique needs of a single person
- ◆ continuity — doing the same things in the same way

Learning Activities

1. Review the health-care plan of ten residents in your facility, and list the different health-care disciplines that have made entries.

2. Explain how the nursing assistant can contribute to the development of the plan of care.

Making factual observation & reporting/recording them accurately.

3. List four ways the health-care plan helps the nursing assistant provide daily care.

(1) Provides specific instructions for care to be given.

(2) Provides necessary info needed prior to giving care.

(3) Provides caregivers w/ the same guidelines

(4) Provides essential data & facts necessary for organizing & planning work.

Notes

Critical Skills Checklist for Chapter 4, Section 1

◆ Accurately complete the Learning Activities. 11/9/00 Date ___ Initial ___

◆ Complete your daily assignment in accordance with the plan of care, and chart resident's response or lack of response to the care provided. Date ___ Initial ___

Date of Completion 11-24-00 Instructor Carolyn Moore, RN

SECTION 2 ■ Organizing Your Time

Objectives

When you have completed this section, you will be able to

- ◆ List the four steps involved in organizing your time
- ◆ Define the term *planning*
- ◆ Place four tasks in the sequence in which they should be completed
- ◆ Write a sample plan for completing your assignment for one day

Key Terminology

- ◆ making rounds — visiting each resident to determine whether he or she has any immediate needs
- ◆ planning — devising a way of getting a job done
- ◆ setting priorities — looking at all of the things that need to be done and putting them in order of what should be done first, second, etc.
- ◆ implement — to start or carry out a plan
- ◆ procrastinating — putting off doing something until some later time

Learning Activities

1. List below the four steps in organizing your time.

   (1) Gathering info

   (2) Planning

   (3) Carrying out the plan

   (4) Revising the plan

2. Define the term *planning*.

Is devising a way of getting the job done

3. Place the following four tasks in the sequence in which they should be performed by numbering each task.

   4 Revising the plan
   1 Gathering information
   3 Carrying out the plan
   2 Developing the plan

4. Write a sample plan for completing your assignment for one day. Follow the plan, and revise it as necessary.

Notes

Critical Skill Checklist for Chapter 4, Section 2

◆ Accurately complete the Learning Activities. 11/9/00 ______ Date ______ Initial

◆ Select a co-worker who consistently completes all work assigned and performs duties with a high level of skill and accuracy. Observe how he or she organizes time. ______ Date ______ Initial

◆ Make rounds with your instructor. Have your instructor verify that care is provided according to the plan of care, that the resident's unit is neat and clean, and that all required documentation is complete. ______ Date ______ Initial

Date of Completion 11-24-00 Instructor Carolyn Moore, RN

SECTION 3 ■ Observation and Charting

Objectives

When you have completed this section, you will be able to

- ◆ Define the term *observation* and explain why it is an important responsibility of the nursing assistant
- ◆ Differentiate between statements that are fact and those that express an opinion
- ◆ List three basic principles of making entries into a resident's health record
- ◆ Identify proper charting principles
- ◆ Match abbreviations and symbols with their definitions
- ◆ Convert standard time to military time

Key Terminology

- ◆ observation — recognizing and noticing a fact or occurrence; paying attention to what is happening around you
- ◆ objective observations — facts you observe that are not distorted by your personal feelings
- ◆ subjective observations — individual judgments about what you observe based on personal feelings

Learning Activities

1. Define the term *observation* and explain why it is an important responsibility of the nursing assistant.

Recognizing & noticing a fact or occurrence.
Not recognizing can be "harmful" It is important because it is planned, careful, & focused.

2. For each of the following, place an *F* by the statements that are factual, and place an *O* by those that are opinions or judgments.

F Mr. Green was up in the wheelchair for one hour.
O Mrs. Smith does not like to take a bath.
O Mr. Brown is mean and nasty.
F Mrs. Green refused her treatments today.
O Mr. Jones's family has abandoned him.
~~F~~ O Mrs. Black has a poor appetite.

3. List three basic principles of making entries into the resident's health record.

(1) Legibility is important

(2) Factuality (legal document)

(3) Brief & exact.

4. Review Figure 4–1. Then identify proper charting principles by auditing the mock charting sample provided by the instructor.

Figure 4–1 Guidelines for charting.

Describe what you see:	
• The activity of the resident, including activities of daily living (dressing, bathing, feeding, personal hygiene, ambulation, continence, etc.)	Describe what kind of assistance is required (total, minimal), and describe what the resident is able to do. Describe how the resident tolerates the activities (is fatigued, short of breath, without difficulty, etc.). Describe the resident's reaction to performing activities of daily living by recording the resident's nonverbal reactions (looks of disgust, shaking fist, uninterested look, etc.).
• The resident's appetite or lack of appetite	Describe what percentage of the food was eaten. If less than 50 percent, list and report what was eaten. For diabetic residents, list and report any food item not eaten. Describe unusual food habits and likes and dislikes (always eats fruit and dessert, never eats meat, is always eating food from other trays, etc.).

Figure 4–1 Guidelines for charting. (continued)

• The resident's body position — how the resident appears while in bed, up in chair, ambulating	Describe contractures or other limitations of movement, posture, gait, special assistive devices (cane, walker, etc.).
• The resident's skin condition, any changes from normal; always refer to the location, size, and special characteristics of any abnormal skin condition	Describe unusual dryness, discolored areas, breaks in the skin, drainage, scratches, or bruises.
• The presence of any abnormal discharge or drainage from any part of the body or present in excretions of the body	Describe the substance, the amount, the color, the odor, and the consistency.
Describe what you hear:	
• The way the resident talks	Describe any difficulties in speaking, special patterns of speech (repetitive words, mumbling, slurred speech, etc.). Describe any differences in how the resident talks to different people (staff, family, friends, etc.).
• What the resident says; ordinary conversations need not be described, but any unusual comments or conversations should be recorded and reported	State exactly what the resident has said that is unusual. Clarify with the resident any statements made to obtain additional information and to avoid misunderstandings or "snap" judgments. If the resident complains of pain, ask and record (1) how and when it occurs, (2) what kind of pain, (3) where it is, and (4) how long it lasts.
• Unusual sounds or noises the resident makes	Describe any unusual coughing, wheezing, gurgling, sounds in the throat, etc.
Describe what you smell:	
• Note changes in the normal odors of the resident's body	Describe unusual odors (fruity, ammonia-like, foul, sour, etc.). Poor personal hygiene can lead to disease and infection. This is easily detected by smell. Bad mouth odor can indicate an infection in the mouth. Drainage from wounds is usually foul-smelling when present.
Describe what you touch:	
• Use your hands to examine the resident and note reactions of the resident to touch	Describe any abnormal areas (smooth, enlarged, swollen, tender, thin, flat, distended, etc.). Notice and describe changes you feel in skin temperature (cold, clammy, hot, dry, etc.). Describe the resident's reactions to touch (painful, no sensation).

Figure 4–2 Commonly used abbreviations.

Time

a.c.	before meals	**a.m.**	morning
p.c.	after meals	**p.m.**	afternoon or evening
q.d.	every day	**h.s.**	hour of sleep (bedtime)
b.i.d.	two times a day	**n.o.c.**	night
t.i.d.	three times a day	**stat**	immediately
q.i.d.	four times a day	**P.R.N.**	as necessary
q.o.d.	every other day	**D/C**	discontinue or stop
q.h.	every hour	$\bar{c}$	with
min.	minute	$\bar{s}$	without

Diagnostic Terms and Body Parts

abd.	abdomen	**nephro**	kidney
ax	axilla	**O.D.**	right eye
Ca	cancer or carcinoma	**O.S.**	left eye
CHF	congestive heart failure	**O.U.**	both eyes
CVA	cerebral vascular accident (stroke)	**osteo**	bone
DX	diagnosis	**psych**	related to psychology
Fx	fracture	**pneumo**	lung
gastric	stomach	**resp**	respirations
G.I.	gastro-intestinal	**Rt**	right
G.U.	genito-urinary	**R.B.C.**	red blood cell
H.O.H.	hard of hearing	**staph**	staphylococcus
Lt	left	**S.O.B.**	short of breath
M.I.	myocardial infarction (heart attack)	**W.B.C.**	white blood cell
N/V	nausea/vomiting		

Measurements

amt.	amount	**lb**	pound
approx.	approximately	**L**	liter
C	Centigrade or Celsius	**min**	minim
cc	cubic centimeters	**mg**	milligram
dr	dran	**no**	number
F	Fahrenheit	**oz**	ounce
g	gram	**ss**	one-half
gr	grain	**tbsp**	tablespoon
gtt	drop	**tsp**	teaspoon
ht	height	**wt**	weight
kg	kilogram	**I, II, III, IV**	one, two, three, four

Treatments

B/p	blood pressure	**Sub-Q**	subcutaneous (injection just into the superficial layers of skin
cap	capsule		
cath	catheter or catheterization	**PT**	physical therapy
C/S	culture and sensitivity (laboratory procedure)	**R**	rectal
		ROM	range of motion
drsg.	dressing	**Rx**	prescription
EEG	electroencephalogram (brain wave tracing)	**S/A**	sugar/acetone (test of urine)

Figure 4–2 Commonly used abbreviations. (continued)

Treatments (continued)

EKG or **ECG**	electrocardiogram tracing of heart function)	**supp**	suppository
Foley	type of urinary catheter	**SSE**	soap suds enema
H_2O	water	**tab**	tablet
H_2O_2	hydrogen peroxide	**TPR**	temperature, pulse, respiration
O_2	oxygen	**TWE**	tap water enema
IM	intramuscular (injection into the muscle)	**U/A**	urinalysis (laboratory procedure)
IV	intravenous (injection into the vein)	**UNG**	ointment
		V/S	vital signs (temperature, pulse, respiration, blood pressure)

Resident Orders and Activity

ADL	activities of daily living	**C/O**	complains of
ad lib	as desired	**Dr.**	doctor
amb	ambulate	**pt**	patient
assist	assistance	**I & O**	intake and output
BM	bowel movement	**NPO**	nothing by mouth
BR	bathroom	**PCP**	patient care plan
BRP	bathroom privileges	**W/C**	wheelchair

5. Complete the crossword puzzle on chart entries in Figure 4–3.

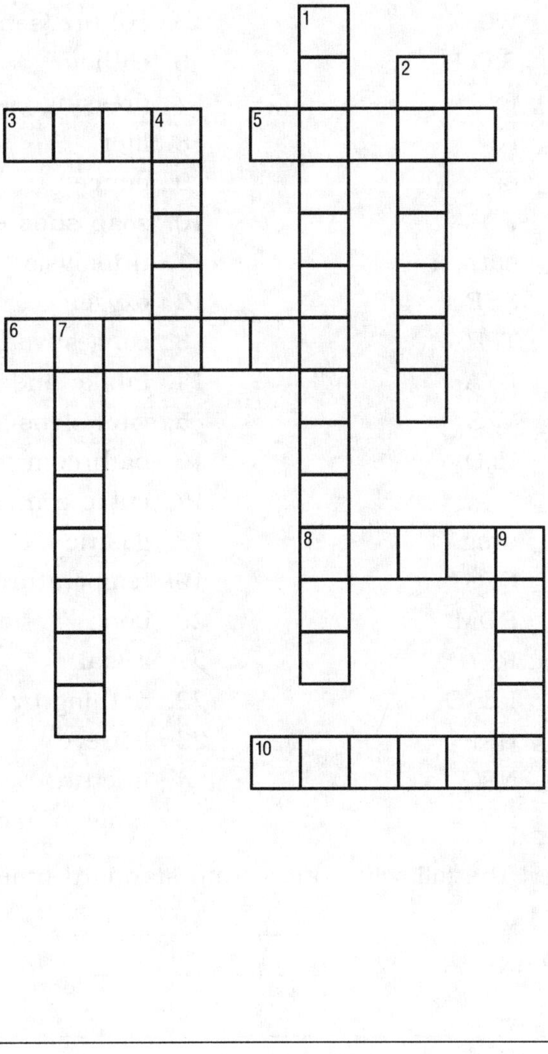

Figure 4–3
Charting crossword puzzle.

Across

3. The entry must be marked with the full, current DAte.
5. Short. – BRieF
6. Based on what has actually happened. Factual
8. The CHARt contains information regarding the resident.
10. All entries should be Signed with first initial, full last name, and title of the person making the entry.

Down

1. In sequence as the event happen – Chronological
2. Able to be read. – Legible
4. Accurate, precise. – EXACT
7. Factual. Accurate
9. To determine when entries are made, all entries should be Timed.

6. Review Figure 4–2. Then match the abbreviations in column A with the definitions in column B.

Column A		Column B
13	CHF	1. white blood cell
23	O.S.	2. short of breath
20	osteo	3. Fahrenheit
18	stomach	4. hydrogen peroxide
1	W.B.C.	5. culture/sensitivity
2	S.O.B.	6. catheter
24	Fx	7. dressing
17	cc	8. liter
9	oz	9. ounce
3	F	10. soap suds enema
6	cath	11. urinalysis
10	SSE	12. oxygen
19	TPR	13. congestive heart failure
11	U/A	14. intake and output
15	V/S	15. vital signs
4	H_2O_2	16. bathroom privileges
12	O_2	17. cubic centimeter
7	drsg.	18. gastric
5	C/S	19. temperature, pulse, respiration
25	ROM	20. bone
21	R	21. rectal
14	I & O	22. nothing by mouth
16	BRP	23. left eye
22	NPO	24. fracture
8	L	25. range of motion

7. Convert the following times from standard time to military time.

a. 10 A.M. 10:00

b. 1 P.M. 13:00

c. 6 P.M. 18:00

d. 12 midnight 00:00\24:00

Notes

Critical Skill Checklist for Chapter 4, Section 3

◆ Accurately complete the Learning Activities. Date 11\9\00 Initial 7f

◆ Prepare a chart on assigned residents using information presented in this chapter, and have your instructor review it for content and accuracy. Date ______ Initial ______

Date of Completion 11-24-00 Instructor Carolyn Moore, RN

SECTION 4 ■ Weight and Vital Signs

Objectives

When you have completed this section, you will be able to

◆ List the necessary criteria for obtaining accurate weights

◆ Weigh a resident using a standing scale

◆ Weigh a resident using a mechanical lift

◆ Weigh a resident using a bed scale

◆ Measure a resident's height using a tape measure

◆ Distinguish between conditions that increase body temperature and those that decrease body temperature

◆ Identify temperature readings that should be reported to the charge nurse immediately

◆ Read sample thermometers accurately

◆ Measure oral, rectal, and axillary temperatures using a glass thermometer

- Measure oral, rectal, and axillary temperatures using a battery-operated electronic thermometer
- Identify four sites on the body where the pulse can be measured
- Distinguish between conditions that increase the pulse and those that decrease the pulse
- Measure a resident's pulse accurately
- Identify different types of respiration
- Measure a resident's respiration accurately
- Identify which reading represents the systolic blood pressure and which gives the diastolic blood pressure
- Identify conditions that cause the blood pressure to increase and those that cause it to decrease
- Measure a resident's blood pressure accurately

Key Terminology

- perpendicular — at a right angle
- vital signs — readings of temperature, pulse, blood pressure, and respiration
- calibrated — marked in degrees and fractions of degrees
- bulb — the portion of the thermometer that is placed in direct contact with the resident's body
- stem — the portion of the thermometer opposite the bulb
- oral — related to the mouth
- rectal — related to the rectum or anus
- axillary — related to the area of the armpit
- pulse — the rhythmic expansion and contraction of the arteries; can be measured to show how fast the heart is beating
- radial pulse — the measurement of the heartbeat at the wrist
- rate — the number of pulse beats per minute
- rhythm — the regularity of the pulse beats
- force — how strong the pulse feels (weak, bounding)
- apical pulse — the measurement of the heartbeat at the apex of the heart
- stethoscope — an instrument used to listen to various sounds in the body, such as heartbeat or breathing sounds
- respiration — the process of inhaling and exhaling
- labored respiration — the respiration of a resident who struggles or works hard to breathe and may make gurgling, rattling, or wheezing sounds
- stertorous respiration — the respiration of a resident who makes abnormal noises, like snoring, when breathing
- abdominal respiration — respiration characterized by using mostly the abdominal muscles

- ◆ shallow respiration — respiration in which only the upper part of the lungs is being used in breathing
- ◆ irregular respiration — respiration in which the depth of breathing changes and the rate of the rise and fall of the chest is not steady
- ◆ Cheyne-Stokes respiration — respiration characterized by irregular breathing; respiration is at first slow and shallow, then becomes faster and deeper, until it reaches a peak and slows again
- ◆ blood pressure — the force of the blood pushing against the walls of the blood vessels
- ◆ systolic pressure — the highest pressure within an artery, which occurs when the heart is contracting
- ◆ diastolic pressure — the lowest pressure within an artery, which occurs when the heart is most relaxed
- ◆ hypertension — a condition in which blood pressure is higher than the normal range for a person's age
- ◆ hypotension — a condition in which blood pressure is lower than the normal range for a person's age
- ◆ sphygmomanometer (also referred to as a *blood pressure cuff*) — an instrument used to measure the blood pressure
- ◆ mercury type — a blood pressure gauge on which the level of a column of mercury on a measuring scale determines the correct blood pressure reading
- ◆ aneroid type — a blood pressure gauge on which a pointer on a dial with a measuring scale determines the correct blood pressure reading

---

Learning Activities

1. To obtain a resident's accurate weight, every effort should be made to weigh the resident at the ___Same___ time of day, with the resident wearing the ___Same___ type or amount of clothing, using the ___Same___ scale.

2. Next to each of the following conditions, write an *I* if the body temperature would be increased or a *D* if the body temperature would be decreased.

   ___I___ Infection
   ___I___ Shivering
   ___D___ Shock
   ___D I___ Dehydration
   ___D___ Age
   ___D___ Aspirin

3. Circle the temperatures listed below that should be reported to the charge nurse immediately.

   a. 100 R
   (b.) 37.6
   c. 99 A
   (d.) 38 R
   (e.) 37.2 A
   f. 98.6
   (g.) 101 R
   (h.) 100

4. Read the thermometers illustrated in Figure 4–4, and record your readings in the spaces provided.

a. 98.2
b. 100.8
c. 96.8
d. ~~100.68~~ 100.6

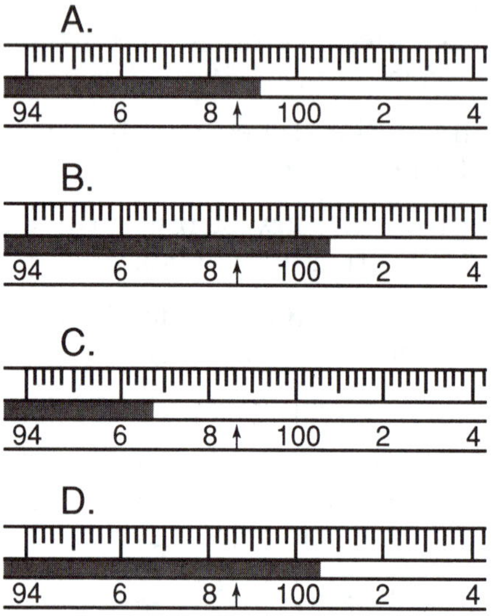

Figure 4–4
Thermometer readings.

5. On the diagram of the body in Figure 4–5, place an asterisk (*) in four places where the pulse can be measured.

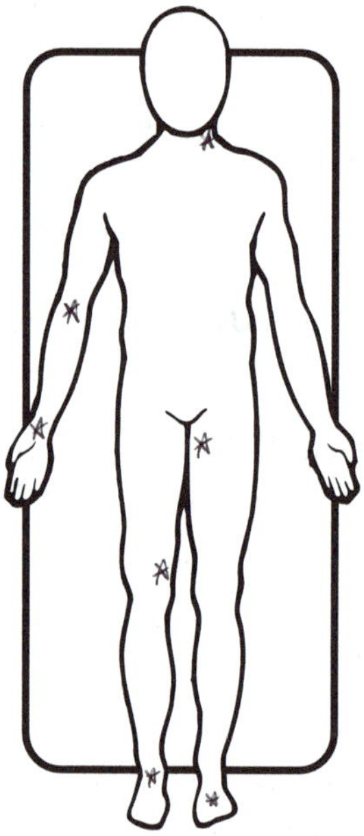

Figure 4–5
Places where the pulse can be measured.

6. Which of the following conditions tend to increase the pulse rate?

a. Sleep
b. Fever
c. Exercise
d. Cold
e. Stress

7. Match the types of respiration in column A with the descriptions in column B.

Column A

C stertorous

A shallow

B Cheyne-Stokes

Column B

a. breathing with only the upper part of the lungs

b. breathing is slow and shallow, then faster and deeper, then slow and shallow again; may even stop

c. abnormal breathing noises like snoring

8. In the blood pressure reading 120/80, 120 represents the Systolic pressure, and 80 represents the Diastolic pressure.

9. Which of the following conditions would cause the blood pressure to increase?

a. Raising the head of the bed

b. Lowering the head of the bed

c. Stress

d. Age

e. Rest

f. Shock

Notes

Critical Skill Checklist for Chapter 4, Section 4

◆ Accurately complete the Learning Activities. 11/9/00 Date Initial

◆ Demonstrate weighing a resident using a standing scale. 11/9 Date Initial

◆ Demonstrate weighing a resident using a mechanical scale. 11/9 Date Initial

- Demonstrate weighing a resident using a bed scale.

  ______ Date ______ Initial

- Demonstrate measuring a resident's height using a measuring tape.

  ______ Date ______ Initial

- Demonstrate measuring oral, rectal, and axillary temperatures using a glass thermometer.

  ✓ Date ______ Initial

- Demonstrate measuring oral, rectal, and axillary temperatures using a battery-operated electronic thermometer.

  ✓ Date ______ Initial

- Demonstrate measuring temperature using an ear-probe thermometer.

  ______ Date ______ Initial

- Demonstrate measuring a resident's pulse.

  11/9 Date TJ Initial

- Demonstrate measuring a resident's respirations.

  11/9 Date TJ Initial

- Demonstrate measuring a resident's blood pressure.

  11/9 Date TJ Initial

Date of Completion 11-24-00 Instructor Carolyn Moore, RN

CHAPTER 5

Anatomy, Physiology, Cancer, and the Senses

SECTION 1 ■ Introduction to Anatomy and Physiology

Objectives

When you have completed this section, you will be able to

- ◆ Explain why it is helpful for the nursing assistant to understand basic principles of anatomy and physiology
- ◆ Define the terms *anatomy* and *physiology*
- ◆ Explain the concept of homeostasis
- ◆ List five basic physical needs
- ◆ Match the parts of a cell with their functions
- ◆ Identify the four components in the organization of the body
- ◆ Identify the various organs of the body

Key Terminology

- ◆ anatomy — the study of body parts, how the body is made, and what it is made of
- ◆ physiology — the study of how the body functions and how the various parts work independently and together
- ◆ anatomic position — body position in which a person is standing straight, facing the examiner, with palms out and feet together; in the study of anatomy, all terms of reference are made in relation to the anatomic position
- ◆ superior — toward the head
- ◆ inferior — toward the feet
- ◆ homeostasis — the body's attempt to keep its internal environment stable or in balance

- cell — the fundamental "building block" of all living organisms
- protoplasm — the substances of which cells are made
- nucleus — the part of a cell that directs its activities, similar to a command center
- chromosomes — threadlike structures within a cell that carry the heredity material
- cytoplasm — the protoplasm outside the nucleus in a cell
- cell membrane — the rim, or edge, of a cell
- metabolism — the work of a cell involving complex processes that use oxygen and give off carbon dioxide
- tissue — a group of the same type of cells functioning in the same way
- organ — a body part consisting of two or more tissues working together to perform a particular function
- system — a group of organs that perform the same function

Learning Activities

1. Explain why it is helpful for the nursing assistant to understand basic principles of anatomy and physiology.

   This knowledge will help w/ understanding why certain kinds of nursing care are necessary.

2. Define the terms *anatomy* and *physiology*.

   Anatomy: Study of body parts, how the body is made, what it is made of

   Physiology: Study of how the body functions, how the body parts work independently & together

3. Explain the concept of homeostasis.

The body's attempt to Keep its internal enviornment stable or in balance.

4. List the five basic physical needs.

(1) Oxygen

(2) Food / fluids

(3) Activity / Rest

(4) PROTETCTION (SHELTER)

(5) ELIMINATION OF BODY WASTES

5. Match the parts of a cell in column A with their functions in column B.

Column A		Column B
B	nucleus	a. work center of the cell
A	cytoplasm	b. command center of the cell
C	cell membrane	c. allows certain materials to pass in and out of the cell

6. The body is organized systematically and includes four basic components. Fill in the missing parts.

a. Cells

b. Tissues

c. Organs

d. Systems

7. The drawing of the male body in Figure 5–1 shows the various organs. Identify them in the spaces provided.

Figure 5–1
Organs of the male body.

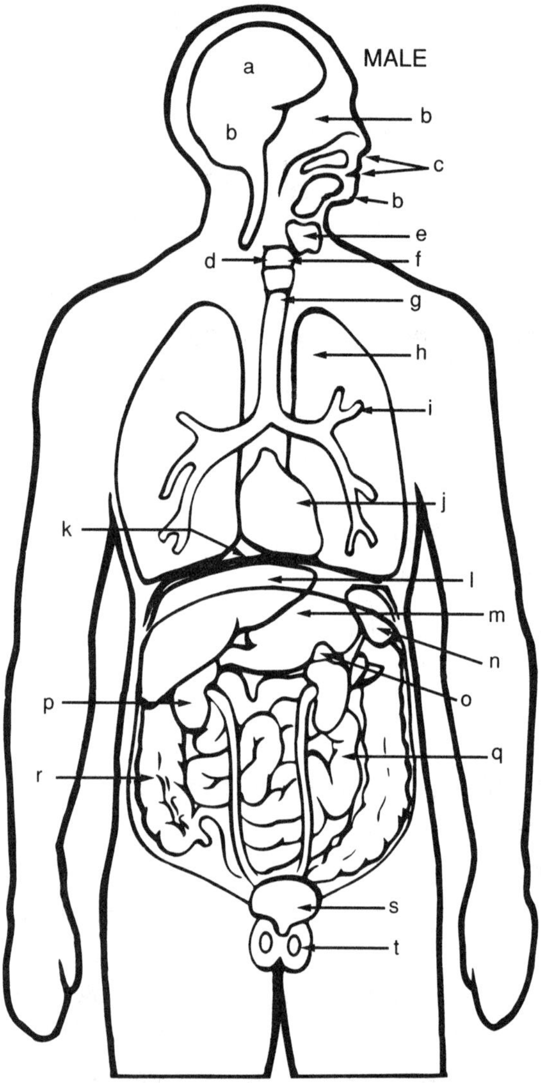

a. Brain

b. Major Sense organs

c. Respatory organs

d. Esophagus

e. Thyroid gland

f. Larynx

g. Trachea

h. Lungs

i. Bronchi

j. Heart

k. Diaphrogm

l. Liver

m. Stomach

n. Spleen

o. Adrenal glands

p. Kidneys

q. Small intestine

r. Large intestine

s. Bladder

t. Reproductive organs

Notes

Critical Skill Checklist for Chapter 5, Section 1

◆ Accurately complete the Learning Activities. 11/9/00 Date TJ Initial

Date of Completion 11-24-00 Instructor Carolyn Moore, RN

SECTION 2 ▪ Cancer

Objectives

When you have completed this section, you will be able to

- ◆ Describe the basic mechanisms of cancer
- ◆ List cancer's seven warning signals
- ◆ Describe the three most common types of cancer treatment

Key Terminology

- ◆ cancer — a form of cellular disorder in which the normal mechanisms of the cell that control the rate of growth, cell division, and movement are disturbed
- ◆ metastasize — to spread to other parts of the body, through blood and lymphatic vessels, where the cancer cells continue to grow
- ◆ carcinoma — a type of cancer most often found in skin and in the lining of hollow organs and passageways
- ◆ sarcoma — a type of cancer most often found in bone, muscle, cartilage, and lymph systems
- ◆ carcinogen — a substance that causes cancer
- ◆ cure — to correct or remove a problem
- ◆ control — to stop or limit growth

- palliation — the relief of symptoms or pain
- surgery — the removal of tissue by means of an operation to cut out diseased parts
- radiation therapy — the use of high-energy waves to stop cancer cells from growing or multiplying
- chemotherapy — the use of drugs or medication to treat the disease
- orally — by mouth
- intramuscularly — by injection into a muscle
- intravenously — by injection into a vein

Learning Activities

1. Describe the basic mechanisms of cancer.

the invasion of tissues + even the spreading to blood or lymphatic vessels. invades the Cell's normal Mechanisms which Control the rate of growth, cell division.

2. List cancer's seven warning signals.

(1) Change in bowel or bladder habits

(2) Sores that don't heal

(3) Unusual bleeding or discharge

(4) Thickening or lump in breast or elsewhere.

(5) Indigestion or difficulty swallowing.

(6) Obvious Changes in wart or mole

(7) Nagging Cough or hoarseness.

3. Describe the three most common types of cancer treatment.

(1) Surgery - Removeal

(2) Radation Therapy - high energy rays.

(3) Chemotherapy - drugs

Notes

Critical Skill Checklist for Chapter 5, Section 2

- Accurately complete the Learning Activities.

11/9/00 Date

TA Initial

Date of Completion 11-24-00

Instructor Carolyn Moore, RN

SECTION 3 ■ Care of the Resident with Cancer

Objectives

When you have completed this section, you will be able to

- List four common side effects associated with radiation therapy and chemotherapy
- List two specific nursing measures that can help reduce side effects or complications
- Describe ways you would like others to provide you with emotional support if you were a cancer victim

Key Terminology

- ◆ fatigue — a condition in which a person becomes tired easily
- ◆ alopecia — loss of scalp and body hair

Learning Activities

1. List four common side effects associated with radiation therapy and chemotherapy.

   (1) Fatigue

   (2) Loss of appetite leading to malnutrition

   (3) Loss of hair

   (4) Emotional stress.

2. List two specific nursing measures that can help reduce the side effects or complications of cancer treatment.

   (1) Be sensetive

   (2) Keep them involved in activities

3. Describe ways you would like others to provide you with emotional support if you were a cancer victim.

   Know they are there for support. Words of comfort & hope. Etc

Notes

Critical Skill Checklist for Chapter 5, Section 3

◆ Accurately complete the Learning Activities.

11/9/00 Date

TY Initial

Date of Completion 11-24-00 Instructor Carolyn Moore RN

SECTION 4 ■ The Senses

Objectives

When you have completed this section, you will be able to

- Describe three types of visual disturbances
- Identify age-related changes in the sense of taste
- Describe how the loss of sensation of temperature and pain can pose a hazard to the safety of elderly residents

Key Terminology

- sensory neurons — specialized types of nerve cells
- stimulus — an action or agent that causes a response in an organ or organism
- presbyopia — a condition of the eye in which the lens loses its ability to focus clearly
- cataract — a condition of the eye in which the lens undergoes changes that decrease its transparency
- glaucoma — a condition of the eye in which pressure within the eye increases
- tympanic membrane — the eardrum
- olfaction — the sense of smell

Learning Activities

1. Match the visual disturbances in column A with the signs or symptoms in column B.

Column A	Column B
B presbyopia	a. pain above the eye, halos around lights
A glaucoma	b. loss of ability to focus clearly, loss of lens elasticity
C cataract	c. cloudy vision

2. The aging process results in a loss of taste, particularly for which two of the following?

   (a.) Sweet
   b. Sour
   (c.) Salty
   d. Bitter

3. The loss of sensation of temperature and pain is common among the elderly. Give examples of how this loss might affect the safety of elderly residents.

Heat - food, water
Cold - hypothermia
Cuts / brusing - not aware

Notes

Critical Skill Checklist for Chapter 5, Section 4

- Accurately complete the Learning Activities. 11/9/00 Date TF Initial

Date of Completion __________ Instructor ____________________

SECTION 5 ■ Problems Related to the Sensory System

Objectives

When you have completed this section, you will be able to

- List four ways the nursing assistant can help prevent sensory deprivation
- Indicate, by using a clock, the location of foods on a tray
- Give four nursing approaches that are appropriate when caring for a blind resident
- Identify correct statements describing the care of the hard-of-hearing resident

Key Terminology

- sensory deprivation — a loss or lack of stimulation from the surrounding world
- unconscious — being unaware of the surrounding environment
- otologist — a specialist in hearing problems and diseases
- hearing aid — a mechanical device used to make certain sounds louder

Learning Activities

1. The nursing assistant can help prevent sensory deprivation in residents by Stimulate the

   (1) Sight - TV - Pictures - mobiles Bulletin Boards

   (2) Hearing - Radio - T.V. Tapes

   (3) Smell - Flowers - Cologne or aftershave

   (4) Taste - offer variety of Foods

   (5) Touch - gentle Touching when care is given. - Hugs - Pats

2. For each food tray pictured in Figure 5–2, give the location of the meat and vegetable, using the clock as a reference.

a. 9 3+4

b. 12 4+5

c. 3 12+6

Figure 5–2
Food trays.

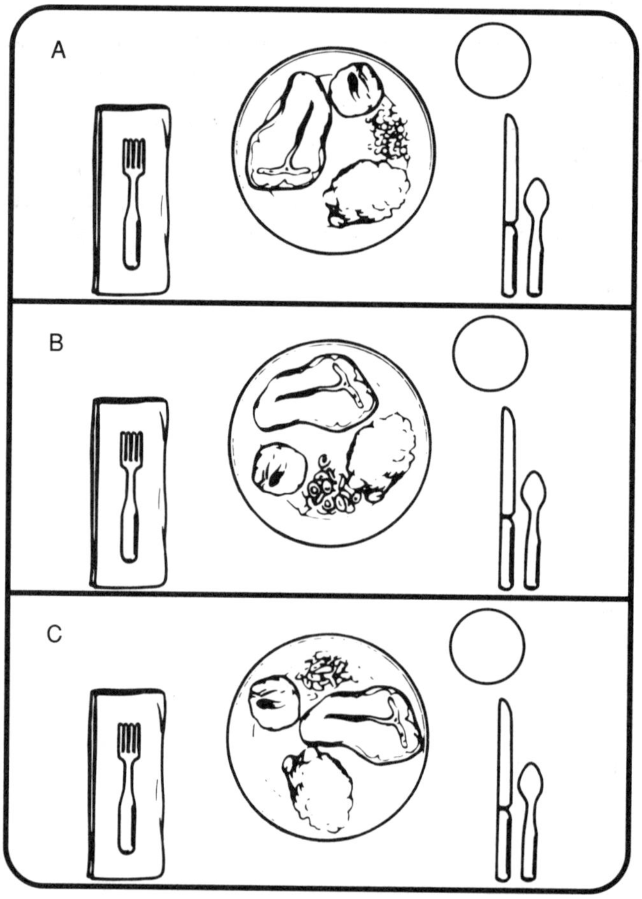

3. When caring for a blind resident, the nursing assistant should do the following.

(1) Identify yourself

(2) Describe what you are doing

(3) Keep residents glasses clean

(4) Describe events occurring (word pic)

4. Indicate which of the following statements about hearing loss are correct (*C*) and which are incorrect (*I*).

__C__ Hearing loss is common after age 65.
__I__ The average resident should have a hearing aid.
__C__ Talking louder does not increase understanding.
__C__ Residents with hearing aids have difficulty hearing in noisy, busy places.

Notes

Critical Skill Checklist for Chapter 5, Section 5

◆ Accurately complete the Learning Activities.	Date ______	Initial ______
◆ Locate the list of residents in your LTC facility who have visual or hearing impairments.	Date ______	Initial ______
◆ Review fire and disaster procedures, and determine the procedures to be followed for the visually or hearing impaired.	Date ______	Initial ______

Date of Completion 11-24-00 Instructor Carolyn Moore RN

CHAPTER 6

The Integumentary System

SECTION 1 ▪ Anatomy and Physiology

Objectives

When you have completed this section, you will be able to

- List four functions of the integumentary system
- Relate changes in skin condition to possible causes
- Explain how the skin helps regulate body temperature

Key Terminology

- epidermis — the outer layer of skin, the visible skin
- dermis — the second layer of skin
- follicle — the root of the hair
- appendage — an attachment usually connected to another body structure
- podiatrist — a foot specialist
- erythema — redness of the skin
- cyanosis — blue or gray color of the skin
- eschar — black or scablike area on the skin

Learning Activities

1. The functions of the integumentary system are

(1) Protect the body

(2) Improve appearance

(3) Regulate body temp

(4) Eliminate waste through sweat

(5) Produce vitamin D when exposed to sun

2. Match the changes in skin condition in column A with the possible causes in column B.

Pg. 153

Column A		Column B
A	redness	a. prolonged pressure, infection, increased body temperature
C	eschar	b. decreased circulation
D	pale or white appearance	c. tissue death
B	cyanosis	d. circulation problems related to shock

3. Explain how the skin helps regulate body temperature.

It reduces body temp. when blood vessels near the skin dialate (becomes larger). This brings more body heat to the skin surface which causes heat to be lost to cooler air. Evaporating perspiration also carries heat away from the skin.

When body heat needs to increase, perspiration stops. Blood vessels contract (smaller) decreasing the heat brought to the surface of the skin.

When we feel cold, we shiver which creates warmth due to muscle activity.

Notes

Critical Skill Checklist for Chapter 6, Section 1

◆ Accurately complete the Learning Activities. 11/9/00 Date ____ Initial

◆ Review the anatomical illustration, "Membranes" (Figure 6-1, p. 152 in the text). ____ Date ____ Initial

Date of Completion 11-24-00 Instructor Carolyn Moore, RN

SECTION 2 ■ Pressure Sores

Objectives

When you have completed this section, you will be able to

- ◆ List the three causes of pressure sores
- ◆ Identify the sites on the body where pressure sores are most likely to occur
- ◆ Identify conditions that increase the risk of developing a pressure sore
- ◆ List five ways the nursing assistant can prevent pressure sores from occurring
- ◆ Describe the correct use of two pressure-sore-prevention devices

Key Terminology

- ◆ pressure sores — sores caused by the death of tissue resulting from a lack of oxygen and nutrients; often referred to as *decubitus ulcers* or *bed sores*
- ◆ pressure points — areas on the body where there is little fat between the skin and the bones
- ◆ shearing — when the skin moves one way while the bone and tissue under the skin move another way
- ◆ anemia — a condition in which there are not enough red blood cells
- ◆ debridement — the removal of dead tissue
- ◆ hydrated — having adequate fluid intake

Learning Activities

1. Pressure sores are caused by Pressure, shearing, and Moisture.

2. Place asterisks (*) on the illustration in Figure 6–1 to show where pressure sores are most likely to occur.

Figure 6–1
Pressure points.

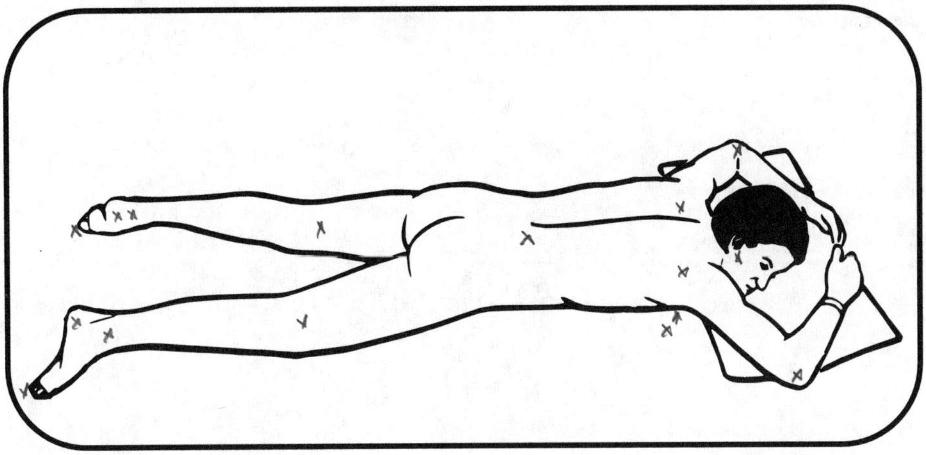

3. Place an X by the conditions below that increase a resident's risk of developing a pressure sore.

_______	Heart disease	_______	Arthritis
__X__	Diabetes	__X__	Overweight
__X__	Anemia	__X__	Underweight
_______	Congestive heart failure		

4. Identify five ways the nursing assistant can help prevent pressure sores.

(1) Keeping skin clean & dry.

(2) Providing lotion

(3) Gentle massage

(4) Keep bed & articles wrinkle free

(5) Keep pt. hydrated.

5. Select two devices from the following list, and describe how they should be used.

a. Eggcrate mattress - Cushions body
b. Sheepskin heel protectors - to keep heels, feet from rubbing against sheets
c. Alternating-pressure mattress - Redistributes weight
d. Foam ring - to be used for pt. to sit on. Pt should reposition as much as possible

Notes

Critical Skill Checklist for Chapter 6, Section 2

- Accurately complete the Learning Activities. 11/9/00 Date ____ Initial ____
- Review the procedures in your facility regarding the use of pressure-reducing devices. Date ____ Initial ____
- Review the documentation requirements when using pressure-reducing devices and when repositioning residents. Date ____ Initial ____
- Using the risk factors identified, determine which of your assigned residents need pressure-reducing devices, and report their names to the charge nurse. Date ____ Initial ____

Date of Completion 11-24-00 Instructor Carolyn Moore RN

SECTION 3 ■ Care of the Skin

Objectives

When you have completed this section, you will be able to

- List three goals of skin care
- Give four reasons for bathing residents

- ◆ Recognize appropriate guidelines for bathing residents
- ◆ Give a complete bed bath
- ◆ Give a back rub
- ◆ Give perineal care
- ◆ Give a tub bath
- ◆ Give a shower

Key Terminology

- ◆ partial bath — the cleansing of only certain areas of the body, usually the face, hands, underarms, and perineal area
- ◆ perennial area — in the female, the area between the vagina and the anus; in the male, the area between the scrotum and the anus

Learning Activities

1. The goals of skin care are to

   (1) provide cleanliness

   (2) promote circulation

   (3) prevent injury

2. Give four reasons residents in an LTC facility need bathing.

   (1) Removes dirt

   (2) eleminates body odors

   (3) stimulates circulation

   (4) gives opportunity to examine for abnormalities.

3. For each of the following statements, place a *T* in front of those that are true and an *F* before those that are false.

   F The most important consideration when bathing a resident is to protect yourself from chills.

   T Soap must be carefully rinsed off the resident to prevent drying of the skin.

   F Privacy is not important in bathing.

   T Bath time is a good time to communicate with the resident.

   F An alert resident may be left alone in the bathtub.

Notes

Critical Skill Checklist for Chapter 6, Section 3

◆ Accurately complete the Learning Activities.	11/9/00 Date	TT Initial
◆ Demonstrate giving a complete bed bath.	✓ Date	Initial
◆ Demonstrate giving a back rub.	✓ Date	Initial
◆ Demonstrate giving perineal care.	✓ Date	Initial
◆ Demonstrate giving a tub bath.	✓ Date	Initial
◆ Demonstrate giving a shower.	✓ Date	Initial

Date of Completion 11-24-00 Instructor Carolyn Moore RN

SECTION 4 ▪ Personal Care and Grooming

Objectives

When you have completed this section, you will be able to

- ◆ List the activities included in personal grooming
- ◆ List three conditions that increase the need for oral hygiene
- ◆ Brush the teeth of a dependent resident
- ◆ Care for dentures

- Indicate which residents should not be given nail care by the nursing assistant
- Trim fingernails or toenails
- Care for a resident's hair
- Shave a resident's beard
- Dress a resident in bed
- Dress a resident who is paralyzed on one side
- Explain the terms *AM care* and *PM care*

Key Terminology

- personal grooming — oral hygiene, care of the nails, care of the hair, shaving, makeup, and dressing
- oral hygiene — care of the mouth, gums, and tongue
- AM care — specific procedures provided early in the morning, before breakfast
- PM care — specific procedures provided in the evening, just before bedtime

---

Learning Activities

1. List five activities included in personal grooming.

   (1) Oral hygiene
   (2) Care of nails
   (3) " " hair
   (4) Shaving
   (5) dressing (also makeup if applicable)

2. Residents will need more frequent mouth care when they are unconscious, receiving Oxygen, or have a fever.

3. Nail care for residents who are diabetic or have Circulation disease should not be given by the nursing assistant.

4. AM care includes

   (1) Providing Bathroom opportunity
   (2) Washing face & hands
   (3) Oral hygene
   (4) Preparing resident for breakfast

5. PM care includes

   (1) B.R. opportunity
   (2) Washing face & hands
   (3) bedtime snack
   (4) oral hygene
   (5) Dressing in sleeping attire
   (6) back rub.

Notes

Critical Skills Checklist for Chapter 6, Section 4

- Accurately complete the Learning Activities. 11/9/00 Date ______ Initial ______
- Demonstrate brushing the teeth of a dependent resident. ✓ Date ______ Initial ______
- Demonstrate caring for dentures. ✓ Date ______ Initial ______
- Demonstrate trimming fingernails or toenails. ✓ Date ______ Initial ______
- Demonstrate caring for a resident's hair. ✓ Date ______ Initial ______
- Demonstrate shaving a resident's beard. ✓ Date ______ Initial ______
- Demonstrate dressing a resident who is in bed. ✓ Date ______ Initial ______
- Demonstrate dressing a resident who is paralyzed on one side. ✓ Date ______ Initial ______

Date of Completion 11-24-00 Instructor Carolyn Moore, RN

SECTION 5 ■ Application of Warm and Cold

Objectives

When you have completed this section, you will be able to

- ◆ Describe the effect of heat and cold on blood vessels
- ◆ Give the appropriate temperatures of different types of heat applications
- ◆ List four safety precautions to be followed when using heat or cold

Key Terminology

- ◆ dilate — to become larger or open
- ◆ contract — to become smaller or close down
- ◆ compress — a localized application
- ◆ soak — immersion of either a localized or a generalized part of the body
- ◆ moist application — an application in which water touches the skin
- ◆ dry application — an application in which no water touches the skin

Learning Activities

1. Heat causes blood vessels to dilate (open), and cold causes them to contract (narrow).

2. Match the heat applications in column A with the temperatures in column B.

Column A	Column B
C warm soak	a. 105 F (40.5 C)
B warm compress	b. 115 F (46.1 C)
A tub bath	c. 100 F (37.8 C)

3. When using heat or cold, the nursing assistant should remember these safety precautions.

   (1) Check temp (application) for right temp.

   (2) Comfortable positioning the patient is important.

   (3) Check residents skin

   (4) dry (by patting) the patient thoroughly

Notes

Critical Skill Checklist for Chapter 6, Section 5

◆ Accurately complete the Learning Activities.

	11/9/00	[illegible]
	Date	Initial

Date of Completion 11-24-00 Instructor Carolyn Moore, RN

CHAPTER 7

The Skeletal System

SECTION 1 ■ Anatomy and Physiology

Objectives

When you have completed this section, you will be able to

- ◆ List four functions of the skeletal system
- ◆ Identify examples of the different types of bones
- ◆ Define the terms *ligament*, *tendon*, *bursa*, and *cartilage*
- ◆ Identify two age-related changes that affect the skeletal system

Key Terminology

- ◆ cranium — the bones of the head
- ◆ vertebrae — the bones of the spine
- ◆ osteocytes — the cells that make up bones
- ◆ joint — an area where one bone connects with one or more other bones
- ◆ ligament — a tough, white, fibrous cord that connects bone to bone
- ◆ tendon — an elastic cordlike structure that connects muscle to bone
- ◆ bursa — a small fluid-filled sac that allows one bone to move easily over another
- ◆ cartilage — a tough gristlelike substance that forms a pad at the end of or between bones
- ◆ scoliosis — an abnormal condition of the spine in which the spine curves in an S shape
- ◆ kyphosis — an abnormal condition of the spine in which the spine curves forward, creating a hunchback

- osteoarthritis — a disease that results in the deterioration and abrasion of joint cartilage, with formation of new bone at the joint surfaces
- rheumatoid arthritis — a disease characterized by painful, stiff, swollen joints, resulting in joint deformities
- fracture — the breaking or cracking of a bone
- dislocation — a disruption of the normal alignment of bones in a joint
- sprain — stretched or torn ligaments or tendons that support a joint
- bursitis — a condition characterized by inflammation of the fluid-filled sac, causing pain on movement
- osteoporosis — a condition in which the bone loses calcium and becomes porous (chalklike), weakening the bone and causing it to break easily

---

Learning Activities

1. List four functions of the skeletal system.

To (1) Protect

(2) Support

(3) Provide leverage

(4) Store vital minerals

2. Match the types of bones in column A with the examples in column B.

Column A	Column B
B long	a. ribs
D short	b. femur
A flat	c. vertebra
C irregular	d. phalanges

3. Match the terms in column A with the definitions in column B.

Column A	Column B
C ligament	a. connects muscle to bone
A tendon	b. fluid-filled sac
B bursa	c. connects bone to bone
D cartilage	d. gristlelike substance that forms a pad between bones

4. Circle the changes in the skeletal system that are considered age-related.

   (a.) Fractures
   (b.) Osteoporosis
   c. Rheumatoid arthritis
   (d.) Loss of bone mass
   e. Scoliosis

Notes

Critical Skill Checklist for Chapter 7, Section 1

◆ Accurately complete the Learning Activities.   11/13/00 Date   TJ Initial

◆ Review the anatomical illustration, "Skeletal System" (Figure 7–1, p.180 in the text).   ______ Date   ______ Initial

Date of Completion 11-24-00   Instructor Carolyn Moore, RN

SECTION 2 ■ The Resident with a Fracture

Objectives

When you have completed this section, you will be able to

◆ Define the term *fracture*

◆ List the three goals of fracture treatment

◆ Identify the causes of common problems for a resident in a cast

Key Terminology

- fracture — the breaking or cracking of a bone
- reduction — the setting of a bone in a proper position to promote healing
- immobilized — unable to move
- traction — the exertion of pull on a limb or area of the body using weights
- countertraction — the exertion of pull in an opposite direction

Learning Activities

1. A fracture is

   The breaking or cracking of a bone

2. The goals of treatment for a fracture are

   (1) Reduction (setting the bone)

   (2) Immobilization - (Casts, pins, nails, screws, etc)

   (3) Rehabilitation

3. Match the common problems in column A for a resident in a cast with their related causes in column B.

	Column A	**Column B**
D	change in skin temperature	a. infection that can develop under a cast
C	swelling	b. swelling that can cause pressure on the nerves
B	numbness and tingling	c. the body's response to a nerve injury
A	foul or musty odor	d. pressure on blood vessels or decreased circulation

Notes

Critical Skill Checklist for Chapter 7, Section 2

- Accurately complete the Learning Activities. 11/13/00 Date ___ Initial
- Review your facility's policies and procedures related to resident falls. ___ Date ___ Initial

Date of Completion 11-24-00 Instructor Carolyn Moore, RN

Section 3 ■ Lifting and Moving

Objectives

When you have completed this section, you will be able to

- Describe four tips for promoting good teamwork
- Move a resident using a lift sheet
- Move a resident up in bed with his or her help
- Turn a resident onto his or her side facing away from you and facing toward you
- Turn a resident using the log-rolling technique
- Identify proper lifting and moving techniques

Key Terminology

- lift or turn sheet — a sheet folded and placed under a resident from the shoulders to the knees to assist with lifting and positioning the resident
- trapeze — a device attached to the bed that allows the resident to use the arms to lift and reposition him- or herself in bed
- log-rolling — a technique for turning a resident that moves the body as one unit, maintaining proper body alignment

Learning Activities

1. Describe four tips for promoting teamwork when lifting and moving residents.

(1) Have things / Be ready before asking for help

(2) Decide who is in charge (usually the person assigned to the pt.)

(3) Review out loud what is going to take place.

(4) Coordinate (count - 1,2,3, lift)

2. Using a classmate or co-worker as a resident, practice each of the skills included in this lesson. Then reverse roles. Describe how it felt to be lifted, moved, and turned. What should the nursing assistant have done differently?

3. Mark an *X* by the photographs in Figure 7–1 that show proper lifting and moving techniques.

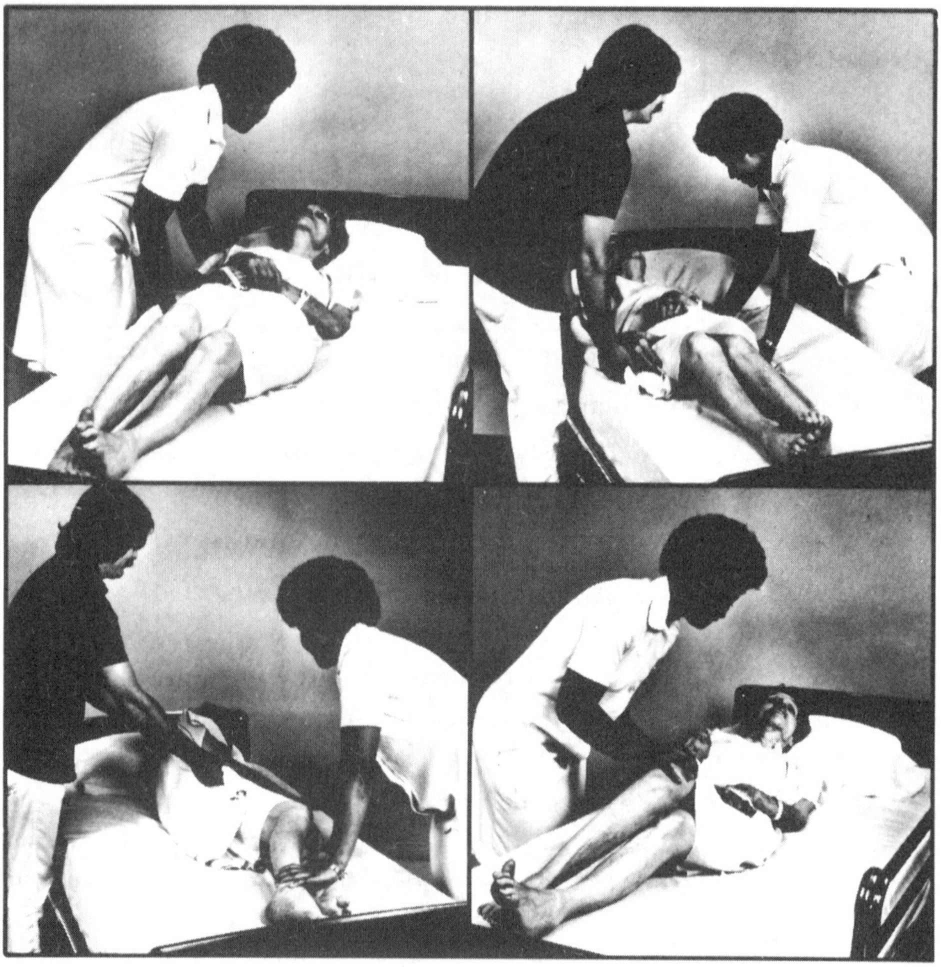

Figure 7–1 Proper and improper lifting and moving techniques.

X

X

Notes

Critical Skill Checklist for Chapter 7, Section 3

◆ Accurately complete the Learning Activities. Date 11/13/00 Initial TJ

◆ Demonstrate moving a resident using a lift sheet. Date ✓ Initial ____

◆ Demonstrate moving a resident up in bed with his or her help. Date ✓ Initial ____

◆ Demonstrate turning a resident away from and toward you. Date ✓ Initial ____

◆ Demonstrate turning a resident using the log-rolling technique. Date ✓ Initial ____

Date of Completion 11-24-00 Instructor Carolyn Moore, RN

SECTION 4 ■ Transfer Techniques

Objectives

When you have completed this section, you will be able to

◆ Transfer a resident using the pivot technique

◆ Transfer a dependent resident

◆ List four principles related to transfer techniques

◆ Distinguish proper transfer techniques from improper ones

Key Terminology

◆ transferring — the process of moving a resident from bed to wheelchair, from wheelchair to toilet, and so on

◆ hemiplegic — paralyzed on one side of the body

◆ transfer belt — a safety belt used to assist with transfers and ambulation

Learning Activities

1. List four principles to be followed when transferring a resident.

(1) Plan and organize before beginning

(2) Encarage the resident to do as much as possible

(3) Use a transfer belt

(4) Use good body mechanics

2. Identify photographs in Figure 7-2 that show correct transfer techniques by marking an X beside them.

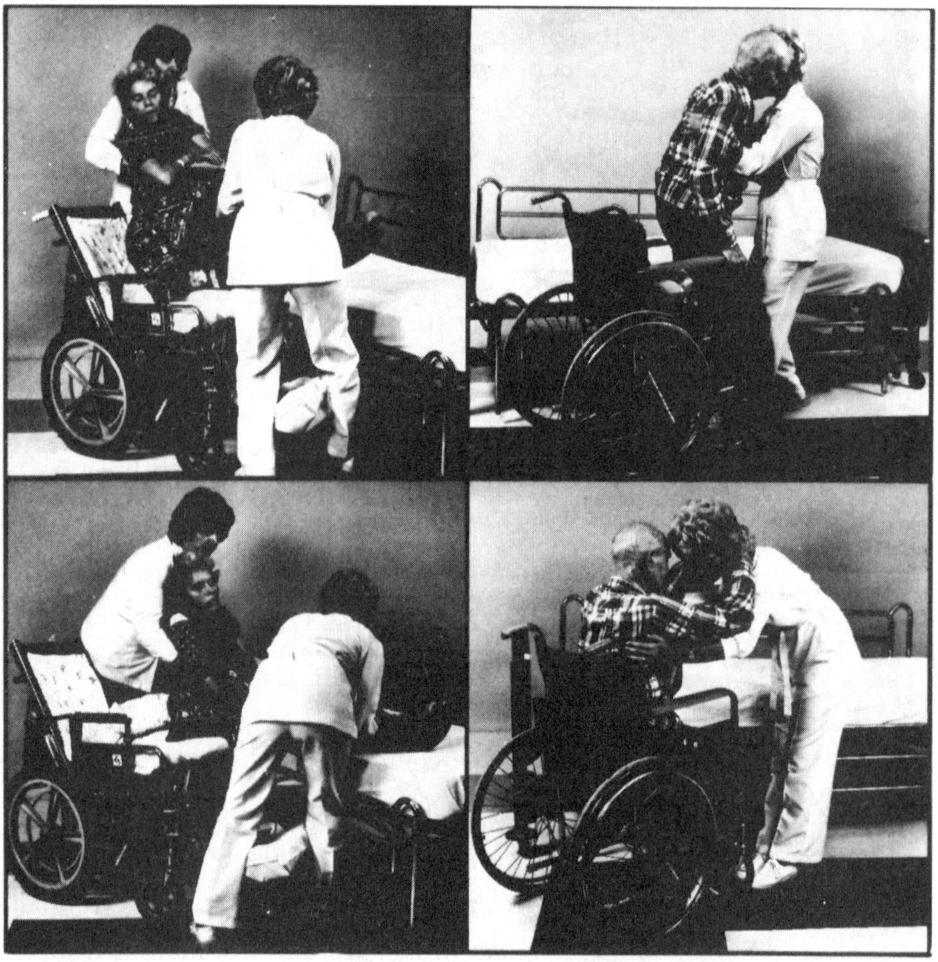

Figure 7–2
Proper and improper transfer techniques.

Notes

Critical Skill Checklist for Chapter 7, Section 4

◆ Accurately complete the Learning Activities.	11/13/00 Date	TJ Initial
◆ Demonstrate transferring a resident using the pivot technique.	✓ Date	Initial
◆ Demonstrate transferring a dependent resident.	✓ Date	Initial

Date of Completion 11-24-00 Instructor Carolyn Moore, RN

CHAPTER 8

The Muscular System

SECTION 1 ■ Anatomy and Physiology

Objectives

When you have completed this section, you will be able to

- ◆ List four functions of the muscular system
- ◆ Define the terms *atrophy*, *contracture*, and *paralysis*
- ◆ Identify the most important nursing measures for preventing or reducing the effects of disuse on the muscular system

Key Terminology

- ◆ striated muscle tissue — a type of voluntary muscle tissue
- ◆ smooth muscle tissue — a type of involuntary muscle tissue
- ◆ cardiac muscle tissue — a type of muscle tissue in the heart that controls heartbeat
- ◆ tendon — an elastic, cordlike structure that connects muscle to bone
- ◆ ligament — a tough, white, fibrous cord that connects bone to bone
- ◆ paralysis — the loss of voluntary movement
- ◆ muscular dystrophy — a progressive muscle disease that causes weakness and atrophy of the muscles
- ◆ multiple sclerosis — a chronic, degenerative disease of the nervous system in which muscles become useless due to damage to the nerves that control them
- ◆ atrophy — decreased muscle mass; wasting of muscle tissue
- ◆ contracture — permanent shortening of the muscle, leading to permanent disability or loss of function
- ◆ ankylosed — a condition in which joints become very stiff, unmovable, and frozen
- ◆ edema — swelling of the joints

Learning Activities

1. The four functions of the muscular system are to provide

   (1) Movement

   (2) Posture

   (3) Protection

   (4) Heat

2. Match the terms in column A with the definitions in column B.

Column A		Column B
B	atrophy	a. inability to move
A	paralysis	b. wasting of muscle tissue
C	contracture	c. shortening of muscle

3. The effects of disuse on the muscular system can be reduced through nursing measures. Identify the three most important measures.

   (1) Range of Motion exercises

   (2) Provide ambulation (walking, moving in an upright position.

   (3) Positioning the pt.

Notes

Critical Skill Checklist for Chapter 8, Section 1

- Accurately complete the Learning Activities. — 11/13/00 Date — TF Initial
- Identify two residents with contractures in your LTC facility and list the ways contractures limit their mobility or function. — ______ Date — ______ Initial
- Review the anatomic illustration, "Types of Muscle Tissue" (Figure 8–1, p. 199 in the text). — ______ Date — ______ Initial

Date of Completion 11-24-00 Instructor Carolyn Moore RN

SECTION 2 ▪ Nursing Care Related to the Muscular System

Objectives

When you have completed this section, you will be able to

- Perform range-of-motion exercises for a dependent resident
- List four observations to be made, reported, and recorded while performing range-of-motion exercises
- List the steps depicting readiness for ambulation
- Ambulate a resident using the step-by-step procedure
- List the safety precautions for ambulation devices
- List four reasons why dependent residents must be repositioned frequently
- Position a dependent resident in a wheelchair
- Position a dependent resident in the supine position, semisupine position, prone position, and semiprone position

Key Terminology

- ambulation — walking or moving about in an upright position
- range of motion — the extent to which a joint can be moved without causing pain
- passive — done for the resident
- active — done by the resident
- adduction — moving an arm or leg toward the center of the body
- abduction — moving an arm or leg away from the center of the body

- extension — straightening an arm or leg
- hyperextension — moving beyond the normal extension
- flexion — bending a joint
- plantar flexion — extending the ankle (toward the sole of the foot)
- dorsiflexion — flexing the ankle (away from the sole of the foot)
- rotation — moving a joint in a circular motion around its axis
- pronation — turning the palm of the hand down
- supination — turning the palm of the hand up
- radial deviation — turning the wrist toward the thumb side of the hand
- ulnar deviation — turning the wrist away from the thumb side of the hand
- gait belt — a belt placed around a resident's waist during ambulation, to give the resident better control over his or her center of gravity
- ambulation device — a device that assists ambulation, such as a brace, cane, crutch, or walker
- alignment — putting in a straight line
- trochanter roll — a rolled towel or blanket placed at the hip joint to prevent external rotation of the leg
- spasticity — an involuntary contracting, or tightening, of the muscle
- bridging — a positioning technique in which support is provided above and below an area

---

Learning Activities

1. List four things that the nursing assistant should observe, report, and record while performing range-of-motion exercises.

   (1) Swollen joints

   (2) Reddened skin over joints

   (3) Weakness

   (4) Complaints of pain on movement

2. Figure 8–1 depicts the four steps for determining the readiness of a resident for ambulation. Identify them.

(1) Their readiness

(2) Strength

(3) Balance

(4) Confidence

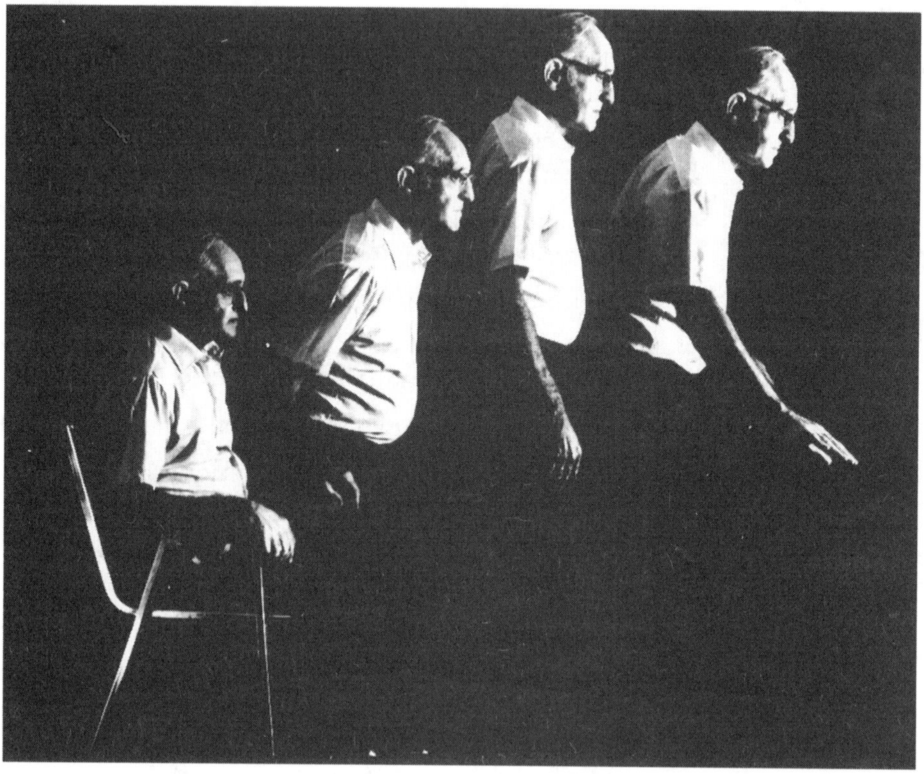

Figure 8–1
Readiness for ambulation.

3. For each of the following ambulation devices, give one safety precaution to be followed by the nursing assistant.

a. Cane Inspect rubber tips

b. Walker also inspect rubber tips for weakness.

c. Brace Observe the skin under brace for irritation

d. Wheelchair Inspect brakes & for torn upholstry

4. If dependent residents are not repositioned frequently, they will be subject to the following problems.

(1) Skin breakdown

(2) Contractures

(3) Pnemonia

(4) Discomfort + Pain

Notes

Critical Skill Checklist for Chapter 8, Section 2

◆ Accurately complete the Learning Activities.	11/13/00 Date	Initial
◆ Demonstrate performing range-of-motion exercises for a dependent resident.	Date	Initial
◆ Demonstrate ambulating a resident using the step-by-step procedure.	✓ Date	Initial
◆ Demonstrate positioning a dependent resident in a wheelchair.	✓ Date	Initial
◆ Demonstrate positioning a dependent resident in the prone and semiprone positions.	✓ Date	Initial
◆ Demonstrate positioning a dependent resident in the supine and semisupine positions.	✓ Date	Initial

Date of Completion 11-24-00 Instructor Carolyn Moore, RN

CHAPTER 9

The Digestive System

SECTION 1 ■ Anatomy and Physiology

Objectives

When you have completed this section, you will be able to

- List the three basic functions of the digestive system
- Label the components of the digestive system
- Match the organs of the digestive system with their functions

Key Terminology

- alimentary tract — the route food takes as it passes from the mouth to the anus
- enzymes — special digestive secretions
- duodenum — the first loop of the small intestine
- bile — a substance, manufactured in the liver and stored in the gallbladder, that has an important function in digestion
- villi — fingerlike projections in the duodenum
- peristalsis — the rhythmic contractions that assist in moving food through the intestines
- appendix — the small projection of tissue located where the large and small intestines meet
- sigmoid colon — the S-shaped lower portion of the large intestine
- feces — semisolid human waste
- rectum — the section of the large intestine immediately adjacent to the outside of the body
- sphincter — a type of muscle that contracts to close a body opening
- ulcer — a cavity that develops and creates an open wound
- gastritis — an inflammation of the stomach
- gallstones — cholesterol crystals that settle out of bile and accumulate in the gallbladder or surrounding ducts

- ◆ hemorrhoids — enlarged, blood-filled vessels that surround the area of the rectum
- ◆ cirrhosis — an inflammation of the tissues of the liver

Learning Activities

1. List the three basic functions of the digestive system.

   (1) Ingest food

   (2) Prepare food for use by the body

   (3) Excrete body waste

2. Label the components of the digestive system in Figure 9–1.

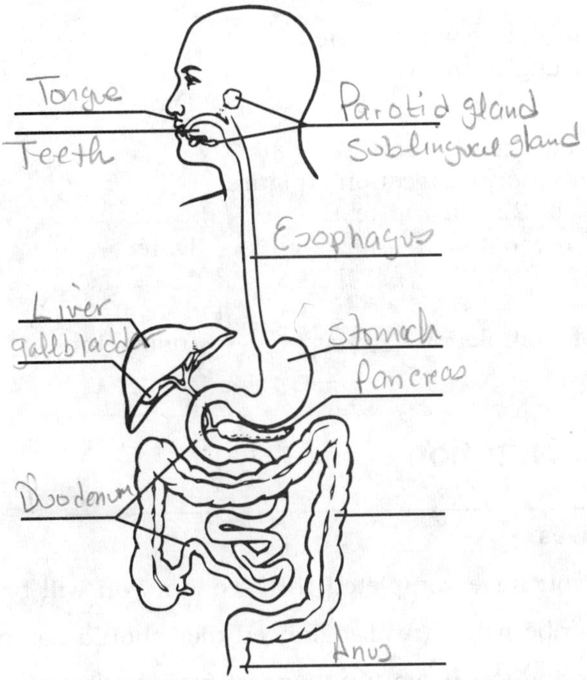

Figure 9–1 Components of the digestive system.

3. Match the organs in column A with the functions in column B.

Column A	Column B
B stomach	a. removes poisons and toxins from the blood
F large intestine	b. mixes food with saliva
A liver	c. absorbs digested food particles
E gallbladder	d. churns and mixes food
D mouth	e. stores bile
C duodenum	f. removes excess water from digested material

Notes

Critical Skill Checklist for Chapter 9, Section 1

- Accurately complete the Learning Activities. 11/13/00 Date TY Initial
- Review the anatomical illustration, "Digestion" (Figure 9–1, p. 221 in the text). ______ Date ______ Initial

Date of Completion 11-24-00 Instructor Carolyn Moore RN

SECTION 2 ■ Basic Nutrition

Objectives

When you have completed this section, you will be able to

- Describe what a well-balanced diet should contain
- Describe the basic functions of carbohydrates, proteins, and fats
- Explain why water is considered an essential nutrient
- List the six food groups of the Food Pyramid and give the recommended number of servings of each per day
- Correctly calculate the percentage of food eaten

Key Terminology

- nutrition — the science of foods and their actions on or relationship to health

Learning Activities

1. What should a well-balanced diet contain?

   (1) Carbohydrates

   (2) Proteins

   (3) fats

   (4) Vitamins

   (5) Iron

   Fluid

2. Describe the basic functions of each of the following:

   a. Carbohydrates Provides energy for work & heat for temp.

   b. Proteins Builds & renews body tissues

   c. Fats also provides work energy & heat energy for maintenance

3. Why is water considered an essential nutrient?

   It provides hydration

   Water Regulates body processes, aids in regulating body Temperature carries Nutrients To Body cells, and carries waste products away from them. Water helps To Lubricate Joints, Water is more immediately Necessary To Life than Food – second only To oxygen.

4. List the six food groups of the Food Pyramid, shown in Figure 9–2, and give the recommended number of servings of each per day.

a. Fats/oils
b. Milk products (Dairy)
c. Meats, poultry, fish, beans, eggs, nuts.
d. Vegetables
e. fruit
f. Grains – Bred, Cerial, rice

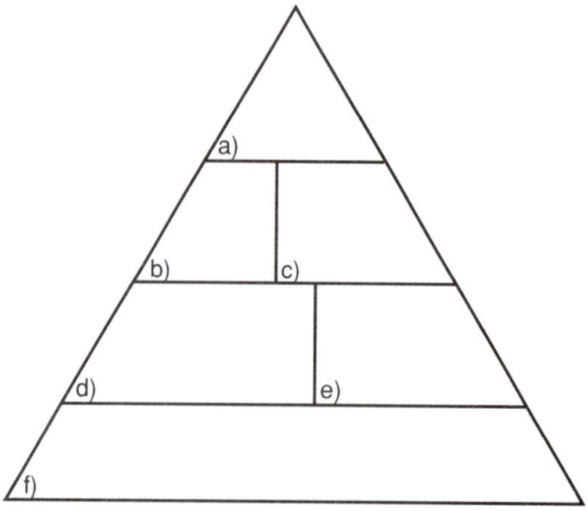

Figure 9–2
The food pyramid.

5. Calculate the percentage of food eaten in the following examples, using the sample charting guide on page 230 of your textbook.

Breakfast:
juice (½ glass) 5
cereal (all) 20
egg (all) 20
toast/margarine (½ slice) 15
milk (½ glass) ~~20~~ 10

Percentage of breakfast = 75%

Lunch
macaroni and cheese (all) 50
peas (½ serving) 2.5
roll/margarine (all) 20
ice cream (all) 10
milk (none) 0

Percentage of lunch = 82.5

Dinner:
baked chicken (½ serving) 20
rice (½ serving) 5
green beans (¼ serving) 1.25
cornbread/honey (all) 20
fruit compote (½ serving) 5
coffee, 1 cup (all) 0
milk (½ glass) ~~15~~ 7.5

Percentage of dinner = 66.25 - 59%

Notes

Critical Skill Checklist for Chapter 9, Section 2

- Accurately complete the Learning Activities. 11/13/00 Date Tf Initial

- Demonstrate calculating the percentage of food eaten on ten different trays, and have your calculations verified by the instructor. ________ Date ________ Initial

- Review the required charting forms for calculating the percentage of food or snacks eaten in your LTC facility. ________ Date ________ Initial

Date of Completion 11-24-00 Instructor Carolyn Moore, RN

SECTION 3 ■ Therapeutic Diets

Objectives

When you have completed this section, you will be able to

- Define the term *therapeutic diet*
- List two ways the nursing assistant can verify a resident's diet order
- Identify the therapeutic purpose of several types of diets
- Explain why it is important for each resident to receive the diet ordered by the physician

Key Terminology

- therapeutic — is effective in the treatment of disease
- hypertension — high blood pressure
- parenterally — receiving nutrition or hydration through a tube inserted into a vein or into the atrium of the heart

- ◆ TPN (total parenteral nutrition) — a system in which a resident receives nutrition intravenously or through a catheter inserted into the atrium of the heart
- ◆ nasogastric tube — a tube inserted through the nose into the stomach
- ◆ gastrostomy tube — a tube inserted surgically directly into the stomach

Learning Activities

1. Define the term *therapeutic diet.*

   a diet designed to assist in the treatment of desease

2. List two ways the nursing assistant can verify a resident's diet order.

   (1) dieit tray Card

   (2) residents Chart

3. Match the diets in column A with the therapeutic purposes in column B.

Column A		Column B
F	low-fat diet	a. for residents who are on a weight-reduction program
D	mechanically altered regular diet	b. for residents who need foods that are easily digested and that avoid irritation of the digestive tract
A	calorie-controlled, low-calorie diet	c. for residents who are hypertensive or who have diseases of the circulatory system or kidneys
E	calorie-controlled, diabetic diet	d. for residents who have difficulty chewing or swallowing
B	bland diet	e. for residents who need a calorie-restricted diet in which food intake is balanced with each resident's insulin requirement and exercise
C	restricted-salt, low-sodium diet	f. for residents who have difficulty digesting fats
G	high-protein diet	g. for residents who have poor intake, who have skin break down, who are seriously debilitated, or who require additional protein to assist in healing and tissue repair

4. Why is it important for each resident to receive the diet ordered by the physician?

There may be certain types of restrictions in the diet, or also things that must be added/needed

(modify/restrict)
Special
Therapeutic
} Diets

Notes

Critical Skill Checklist for Chapter 9, Section 3

- Accurately complete the Learning Activities. — Date: 11/13/00 — Initial: [initials]
- Check the tray cards and health-care plans of four residents, and compare them with the physician's orders. — Date: ______ — Initial: ______
- Determine whether arm bands or tray cards are color-coded in your LTC facility. If so, identify which colors are used for specific diets. — Date: ______ — Initial: ______
- Demonstrate fastening an internal feeding tube to a resident's clothing. — Date: ______ — Initial: ______

Date of Completion 11-24-00 Instructor Carolyn Moore, RN

SECTION 4 ■ Preparing for Mealtime, Serving, and Assisting with Eating

Objectives

When you have completed this section, you will be able to

- List three ways to prepare the resident's environment for mealtime and to prepare the resident for mealtime
- Explain why it is important for residents to eat in the dining area
- Describe how the nursing assistant can be certain of serving the right tray to the right resident
- Feed a dependent resident
- Describe the role of the occupational therapist consultant

Key Terminology

- nutritional supplement — a high-protein drink given to residents who are debilitated or who have poor dietary intake; may be referred to as *nourishments* in some LTC facilities

Learning Activities

1. List three ways to do each of the following.

   a. Prepare the resident's environment for mealtime

   (1) Remove unnecessary supplies or equipment

   (2) " " unsightly & odor producing items

   (3) Adjust lighting

   b. Prepare the resident for mealtime

   (1) Assist with washing hands, brushing teeth, washing face, etc

   (2) Position the patient into the supine position

   (3) Provide opportunity for resident to use toilet, bedpan, urinal, etc before meal.

2. Why is it important for residents to eat in the dining area?

   To provide & encourage for a social time

3. How can the nursing assistant be certain of serving the right tray to the right resident?

By checking the arm band & diet card for comparison

4. Describe the role of the occupational therapist consultant.

Evaluate & works with residents who require special assistance in performing ADL. Also assists the staff in learning help thept. w/ special assistive devices.

Notes

Critical Skill Checklist for Chapter 9, Section 4

- Accurately complete the Learning Activities. 11/13/00 Date TJ Initial
- Demonstrate feeding a dependent resident. ✓ Date ______ Initial
- Volunteer to be fed blindfolded by a fellow nursing assistant. Experience what it is like to not be told which foods are being offered, to be fed too fast, and to be fed without conversation. ______ Date ______ Initial

◆ Determine the procedure followed in your LTC facility if a resident refuses a meal and a substitution is necessary.

Date	Initial

◆ Review facility policies for serving and charting nutritional supplements and between-meal snacks.

Date	Initial

Date of Completion 11-24-00 Instructor Carolyn Moore, RN

SECTION 5 ■ Elimination

Objectives

When you have completed this section, you will be able to

- ◆ Define the term *defecation*
- ◆ List four important observations related to bowel elimination
- ◆ Describe why the accurate recording of a resident's bowel function is essential
- ◆ List three nursing measures used to decrease constipation in the elderly or chronically ill
- ◆ Identify one complication related to constipation that requires the immediate attention of a licensed nurse
- ◆ Insert a rectal suppository
- ◆ Administer a cleansing enema
- ◆ Define the term *colostomy*
- ◆ Change a colostomy bag
- ◆ Collect a stool specimen
- ◆ List four ways the nursing assistant can help a resident regain bowel control

Key Terminology

- ◆ defecation — the process of eliminating waste material from the bowel
- ◆ feces — solid human waste (bowel movement, stool)
- ◆ diarrhea — semifluid feces
- ◆ constipation — a buildup of fecal matter in the large intestine that is not easily passed through the rectum
- ◆ fecal impaction — a serious complication of constipation that blocks the intestine

- enemas until clear — no solid fecal material is present when the solution is expelled
- laxative — medication that loosens the bowel and encourages evacuation
- suppository — medication molded in a cone shape for insertion into the anus
- enema — the introduction of fluid into the rectum and colon to stimulate the bowel to evacuate its contents
- ostomy — a surgical opening on the surface of the abdomen
- stoma — the actual opening of an ostomy
- colostomy — an opening into the colon
- ileostomy — an opening into the ileum
- ureterostomy — an opening into one of the ureters

Learning Activities

1. Define the term *defecation*.

The process of eliminating waste material from the bowel.

2. List four important observations related to bowel elimination.

(1) Changes in color of the stool

(2) Changes in bowel habits

(3) diarrhea / constipation

(4) Presence of Parasites

3. Why is the accurate recording of a resident's bowel function essential?

To Enable Nurse To determine the Resident's Need For Laxative medication

Prevent

4. List three nursing measures used to decrease constipation in the elderly or chronically ill.

(1) ~~Suppository~~ Adequate intake of Food & Fluids

(2) ~~Tapwater enema~~ Exercise & ambulation

(3) ~~Commercially prepared enema~~ Privacy when Toileting

5. One complication of constipation that requires the immediate attention of a licensed nurse is fecial impaction.

6. A colostomy is

an opening into the colon

7. List four ways the nursing assistant can assist a resident regain bowel control.

(1) Encourage the resident to consume adequate amounts of food + fluids.

(2) Report signs of constipation - so medication can be administered.

(3) Answer call light promptly & assist resident w/ the use of bathroom + bed pans

(4) Praise the resident

Notes

Critical Skill Checklist for Chapter 9, Section 5

◆ Accurately complete the Learning Activities.	11/13/00 Date	TJ Initial
◆ Demonstrate inserting a rectal suppository.	— Date	Initial
◆ Demonstrate administering a cleansing enema.	— Date	Initial
◆ Demonstrate changing a colostomy bag.	— Date	Initial
◆ Demonstrate collecting a stool specimen.	— Date	Initial
◆ Review the reporting and documentation procedures of your LTC facility related to residents' bowel function.	Date	Initial

Date of Completion 11-24-00 Instructor Carolyn Moore, RN

CHAPTER 10

The Urinary System

SECTION 1 ■ Anatomy and Physiology

Objectives

When you have completed this section, you will be able to

- ◆ List three important functions of the urinary system
- ◆ Label the components of the urinary system
- ◆ Identify the average adult urinary output for a twenty-four-hour period
- ◆ List three common age-related changes affecting the urinary system
- ◆ List three factors contributing to the development of urinary tract infections

Key Terminology

- ◆ kidneys — bean-shaped organs, lying just below the diaphragm and posterior abdominal wall on either side of the lumbar region of the spine, that remove waste products from the body by producing urine
- ◆ nephrons — microscopic filtering units of the kidneys
- ◆ renal artery — the source from which blood enters the kidneys
- ◆ glomerulus — a network of capillaries in the kidney that filters blood
- ◆ renal pelvis — a collecting funnel from which urine is passed into the right and left ureters
- ◆ ureters — tiny tubes that start at the renal pelvis and empty urine into the bladder
- ◆ stretch receptors — nerve cells in the walls of the bladder that become stimulated when the bladder is full
- ◆ urination — emptying the bladder
- ◆ urethra — the tube leading from the bladder to the outside of the body
- ◆ urinary incontinence — the inability to control urination
- ◆ indwelling catheter — a tube inserted into the bladder that drains urine into a collection bag

- calculi — stones in the kidney or bladder
- frequency — the need to urinate often
- urgency — the immediate need to urinate
- nocturia — waking at night to urinate

Learning Activities

1. Three important functions of the urinary system are the

   (1) Remove wastes from bloodstream

   (2) Produces urine

   (3) Maintain homeostasis

2. In Figure 10–1, label the components of the urinary system.

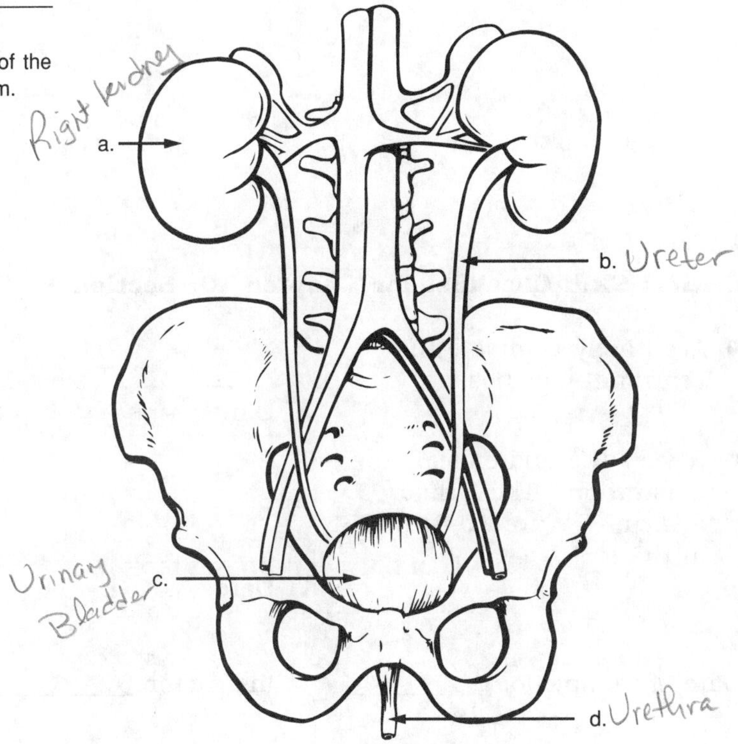

Figure 10–1
Components of the urinary system.

3. What is the average adult urinary output for twenty-four hours?

   a. 1 pint
   b. 2 quarts
   c. 1 gallon
   d. 1½ quarts

4. Name three common age-related changes that affect the urinary system.

   (1) Decrease in muscle tone.

   (2) Amount of urine the bladder holds is decreased.

   (3) Unaware of the need to urinate until bladder is almost full.

5. Three factors contributing to the development of urinary tract infections are

(1) indwelling Catheter / Confined to bed

(2) Incomplete emptying of bladder

(3) Bad hygiene practices

Notes

Critical Skill Checklist for Chapter 10, Section 1

- Accurately complete the Learning Activities. — Date: 11/13/00 — Initial: [initials]

- Review the anatomical illustration, "The Urinary System" (Figure 10–1, p. 252 in the text). — Date: 11/13/00 — Initial: [initials]

Date of Completion 11-24-00 Instructor Carolyn Moore RN

SECTION 2 ■ Fluid Balance—Intake and Output

Objectives

When you have completed this section, you will be able to

- Describe what is meant by *fluid balance*
- Identify the items that should be calculated as fluid intake
- Compute intake accurately
- Compute output accurately
- List three ways the nursing assistant can help residents meet their fluid needs

Key Terminology

- ◆ fluid intake — the amount of fluid consumed by mouth, through special feeding tubes, or through a vein
- ◆ parenteral — into a vein or under the skin
- ◆ fluid output — the amount of fluid eliminated from the body
- ◆ emesis — vomiting
- ◆ hemorrhage — bleeding
- ◆ fluid balance — when the amounts of fluid taken in and eliminated are equal
- ◆ fluid imbalance — when the amounts of fluid taken in and eliminated are not equal
- ◆ edema — swelling due to the accumulation of fluid in joints, tissues, or organs
- ◆ dehydration — a condition in which fluid output is greater than fluid intake
- ◆ central line — a catheter placed into the atrium of the heart
- ◆ calibrated — marked with measurements
- ◆ force fluids — to encourage the intake of oral fluids
- ◆ dialysis — the use of a machine to perform the basic functions of the kidney
- ◆ NPO — nothing by mouth

Learning Activities

1. *Fluid balance* means that the amount of fluids taken in is equal to the amount of fluids eliminated.

2. Circle the items in the following list that should be included as fluid intake.

a. Ice cream	f. Tea
b. Soup	g. Scrambled eggs
c. Jello	h. Cooked cereal
d. Crackers	i. Water
e. Tuna salad	

3. From the following list of items, calculate the resident's fluid intake in cubic centimeters.

Breakfast:	½ 4-oz glass of orange juice 60
480	1 6-oz cup of coffee 180
	2 scrambled eggs
	1 slice of toast with jelly
	1 8-oz glass of water 240
Lunch:	1 8-oz bowl of soup 240
540	1 ham and cheese sandwich
	1 4-oz bowl of jello 120

1 6-oz cup of coffee 180
1 small serving potato salad

Afternoon snack: 1 6-oz glass of juice 180

Dinner: 1 4-oz serving of roast beef
1 serving potatoes/gravy
1 serving green beans
1 serving green salad/dressing
1 6-oz cup of coffee 180
1 4-oz serving ice cream 120
1 slice of bread with butter
1 8-oz glass of water 240

540

2,160 cc's

Evening snack: 1 8-oz glass of milk 240
2 graham crackers

240

Night: 1 6-oz glass of water 180

180

4. From the following list, compute the resident's output for the twenty-four-hour period described. Record the output in cubic centimeters.

7–3 shift	500 cc
3–11 shift	850 cc
11–7 shift	650 cc
Total twenty-four-hour output	2,000

5. The nursing assistant can help residents meet their fluid needs by doing these things.

(1) Offer fluids each time you enter the room

(2) find out what type of fluids they prefer

(3) Have the family assist in encouragement of fluid intake.

Notes

Critical Skill Checklist for Chapter 10, Section 2

- Accurately complete the Learning Activities. 11/13/00 Date ___ Initial ___

- Measure the food containers commonly used in your LTC facility, and make a chart showing the number of cc's in each one. Date ___ Initial ___

Date of Completion 11-24-00 Instructor Carolyn Moore, RN

SECTION 3 ■ Nursing Measures Related to the Urinary System

Objectives

When you have completed this section, you will be able to

- Place a resident on a bedpan and offer a urinal to a male resident
- Give perineal care to a resident with a catheter
- Identify four common places where bacteria can enter the urinary drainage system
- Describe the procedure for collecting a "clean-catch" urine specimen.

Key Terminology

- closed urinary drainage system — a method of eliminating urine from the body through an indwelling catheter, drainage tube, and collection bag, which remain connected at all times; all parts of the system are changed at the same time
- indwelling catheter or foley — a flexible tube that is inserted into the bladder by a licensed nurse and is held in place by an inflatable balloon; urine drains through the catheter and tubing into a collection bag
- reflux — when urine goes from the tubing or collection bag back into the bladder; caused by raising the bag and tubing above the level of the bladder
- midstream clean-catch — a method of obtaining a urine specimen that is free from contamination
- clean-catch — urine that is not contaminated by anything outside the resident's body

Learning Activities

1. In Figure 10–2, indicate four common places where bacteria can enter the urinary drainage system.

Figure 10–2
Urinary drainage system.

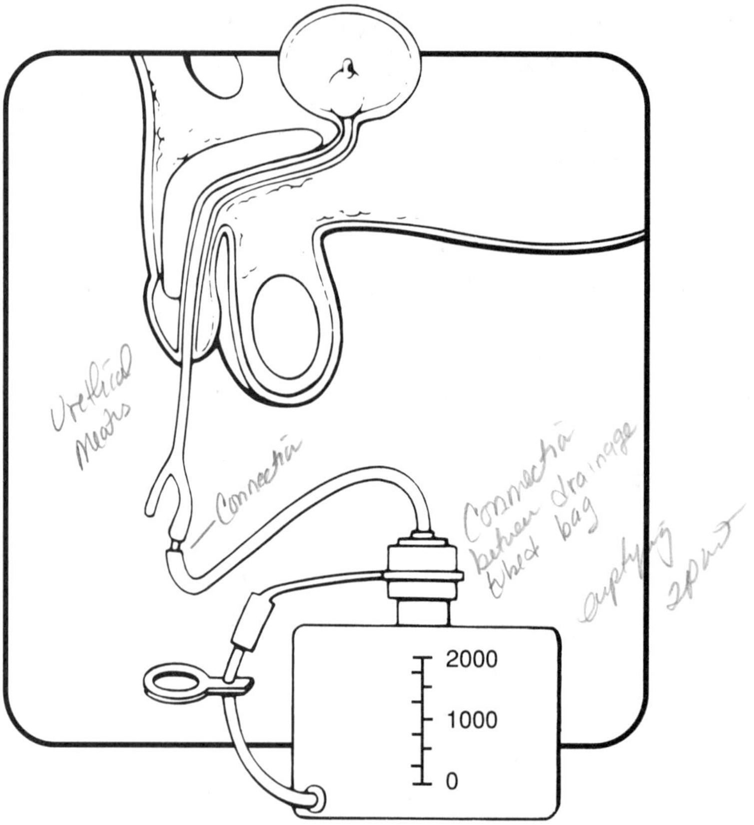

2. To obtain a clean-catch urine specimen, careful __Cleaning/washing__ of the area __of the perineal__ is required. In addition, the specimen is collected in a container that is free of __Contamination__.

Notes

Critical Skill Checklist for Chapter 10, Section 3

◆ Accurately complete the Learning Activities. 11/13/00 Date 1f Initial

◆ Demonstrate placing a resident on a bedpan. ✓ Date ______ Initial

◆ Demonstrate offering a urinal to a male resident ✓ Date ______ Initial

◆ Demonstrate giving perineal care to a resident with a catheter. ✓ Date ______ Initial

Date of Completion 11-24-00 Instructor Carolyn Moore, RN

SECTION 4 ■ Care of the Incontinent Resident

Objectives

When you have completed this section, you will be able to

◆ Define the term *incontinence*

◆ List four possible causes of urinary incontinence

◆ Describe the proper use of disposable briefs

◆ List four nursing measures that can increase a resident's chance of successful bladder retraining

Key Terminology

◆ incontinence — the lack of voluntary control of the bowel, bladder, or both

◆ briefs — disposable or cloth underwear designed to collect the urine or feces of an incontinent resident

◆ bladder retraining — a systematic and individualized method of assisting an incontinent resident to regain control of bladder function

Learning Activities

1. Define the term *incontinence*.

Lack of Voluntary Control of the Bowel, Bladder or Both.

2. List four of the possible causes of urinary incontinence.

(1) Stress/worry

(2) Urinary tract infection

(3) Medications

(4) Confusion

3. Describe the proper use of disposable briefs by filling in the blanks in the following statements.

a. Use disposable briefs only for residents who cannot be toileted/bladder retrained or are unable to use a bedpan.

b. Always select the appropriate size.

c. Check the resident often to see if changing is needed.

d. Observe the skin for any signs of irritation, and report your observations promptly.

e. Dispose of the briefs in the proper container, not in the trash container in the resident's room.

4. List four measures that the nursing assistant can take to increase the resident's chance of successful bladder retraining.

(1) Maintain adequate fluid intake

(2) Answer the call light promptly.

(3) Follow the established plan

(4) Don't give up - it takes time

Notes

Critical Skill Checklist for Chapter 10, Section 4

◆ Accurately complete the Learning Activities. 11/13/00 (Date) TJ (Initial)

Date of Completion 11-24-00 Instructor Carolyn Moore, RN

CHAPTER 11

The Nervous System

SECTION 1 ■ Anatomy and Physiology

Objectives

When you have completed this section, you will be able to

- Describe two functions of the nervous system
- Briefly explain how damage or disease of the nervous system differs from damage or disease of other body systems
- Give the primary function for each of the four areas of the brain
- Explain the basic function of the spinal cord

Key Terminology

- neurons — specialized cells of the nervous system
- cerebrum — the largest portion of the brain, located in the upper portion of the skull
- hemisphere — one-half of the brain; the brain is divided into two hemispheres, right and left
- diencephalon — the area of the brain where the hypothalamus is located
- cerebellum — the part of the brain that coordinates voluntary movement
- midbrain, pons, and medulla — the primary pathways through which nervous impulses reach the brain from the spinal cord
- spinal cord — the long cable of nerves that extends from the area below the medulla to the level of the second or third lumbar vertebra
- reflexes — automatic responses of the muscles or skin to stimulation
- vertebral column — the series of bones surrounding the spinal cord
- autonomic nervous system — the part of the nervous system that supplies the structures and organs of the body that are not under voluntary control

- sympathetic division — the part of the autonomic nervous system that activates the fight-or-flight response during stress, danger, excitement, or illness
- parasympathetic division — the part of the autonomic nervous system that helps conserve energy and is in control during sleep and relaxation

Learning Activities

1. Which two of the following are functions of the nervous system?
   a. To maintain body posture
   (b.) To maintain a balance among all body activities
   c. To protect the body from harm
   d. To nourish the cells of the body
   (e.) To receive signals from inside and outside the body and to relay these signals to and from the brain

2. Damage or disease of the nervous system differs from damage or disease of other body systems because cells within the nervous system called neurons do not have the ability to reproduce or to receive signals when injured.

3. Give the primary function for each of the four areas of the brain.
   a. Occipital lobe the place where what you see is interpreted

   b. Frontal lobe the primary area of thought, reason, & speech

   c. Temporal lobe – the auditory (hearing) area

   d. Parietal lobe the area of awareness of sensation of heat, cold, touch, pressure, & pain.

4. The basic function of the spinal cord is to relay messages to and from the brain and to serve as the center for reflex activity.

5. The word-search puzzle in Figure 11–1 includes key terminology from this section of the text. Find the following words in the puzzle, and circle them.

Figure 11–1 Nervous system word-search puzzle.

M	A	B	V	E	R	T	E	B	R	A	L	C	O	L	U	M	N	C	R	A	F	P	Z	Q
Z	E	X	T	R	V	P	N	L	J	H	F	D	A	T	S	R	Q	P	O	N	S	L	K	J
B	O	D	B	D	F	H	J	B	R	T	H	B	F	M	J	V	E	R	N	I	J	M	C	C
N	A	C	U	E	G	O	C	L	V	P	E	I	G	K	E	Z	X	H	X	L	E	N	E	Y
L	O	P	O	L	M	D	N	L	X	D	M	K	J	D	R	I	A	G	S	T	R	N	R	O
J	C	E	R	E	L	A	T	S	P	U	I	B	L	T	L	H	F	W	S	T	Y	P	E	Q
H	Q	S	P	E	R	A	T	U	Y	Q	S	E	C	N	E	B	D	Y	C	E	G	Z	B	F
F	A	Z	F	Q	W	X	W	V	R	T	P	N	F	I	O	P	S	R	E	D	K	X	R	C
D	C	G	B	D	R	E	G	F	X	R	H	A	B	D	J	S	A	Z	X	I	Y	N	U	P
B	H	I	J	K	L	S	N	A	O	A	E	P	Q	R	U	T	U	V	P	E	C	K	M	N
A	P	O	I	N	N	F	T	L	Q	P	S	R	V	O	A	H	A	X	T	N	S	Q	R	A
N	A	Q	K	O	E	G	L	I	P	S	P	I	V	K	O	T	K	M	X	C	P	C	B	G
I	R	B	L	D	T	P	M	J	V	P	H	R	K	J	L	V	T	K	Q	E	B	M	N	T
A	S	U	C	V	C	N	N	X	Y	I	E	J	K	M	K	U	P	Y	K	P	F	E	L	I
R	C	B	A	E	N	E	U	R	O	N	R	H	I	L	S	V	T	Y	G	H	V	D	K	J
B	D	E	M	L	F	G	H	I	C	A	E	X	M	N	R	W	H	X	H	A	L	O	M	Q
D	P	O	N	K	J	I	M	I	D	L	C	N	C	E	R	E	B	E	L	L	U	M	S	N
I	Q	S	R	G	E	H	M	B	T	C	O	E	Q	Y	P	M	K	I	E	O	M	U	D	Y
M	W	X	D	Z	F	O	A	V	W	O	E	D	Y	Q	P	I	E	R	J	N	N	I	C	K
Y	W	C	O	Y	N	N	A	K	P	R	J	E	N	N	Y	A	N	D	M	A	R	Y	B	L
A	K	E	M	O	T	Y	T	N	I	D	K	K	I	C	O	N	N	I	E	R	A	L	P	H
G	P	R	T	K	A	T	H	Y	K	E	L	L	Y	S	E	X	E	L	F	E	R	U	X	P
K	L	U	E	W	I	S	O	M	A	T	T	P	P	E	R	L	J	U	D	Y	P	R	O	M
L	A	M	N	V	T	O	Q	S	Y	P	R	T	W	V	P	M	N	R	E	W	Q	Y	U	M

Medulla
Cerebrum
Midbrain
Pons
Reflexes
Spinal cord
Cerebellum
Vertebral column
Diencephalon
Autonomic nervous system
Neuron

Notes

Critical Skill Checklist for Chapter 11, Section 1

- Accurately complete the Learning Activities. Date: 11/14/00 Initial: [illegible]

- Review the anatomical drawings of the nervous system (Figures 11–1, 11–2, and 11–3, pp. 274 and 275 in the text). Date: ______ Initial: ______

Date of Completion 11-24-00 Instructor Carolyn Moore, RN

SECTION 2 ▪ The Resident with a Nervous System Abnormality

Objectives

When you have completed this section, you will be able to

- List three common symptoms of Parkinson's disease
- Describe the nursing care of a resident with Parkinson's disease
- Identify the age group most often affected by multiple sclerosis
- Describe why the nature of multiple sclerosis makes adjustment difficult for the victim
- Define the terms *remission* and *exacerbation* in relation to multiple sclerosis
- Define the terms *paraplegic* and *quadriplegic*
- Give examples of how spinal cord injury affects each of the body systems
- Describe the measures to be taken when autonomic dysreflexia occurs

- Explain the nature of a cerebrovascular accident
- Select a stroke victim and write a case study
- List four tips for improving communication with an aphasic resident
- Describe three goals of nursing care for a resident with impaired consciousness
- Identify five conditions that increase the frequency of seizures
- Identify true and false statements about epilepsy
- Describe the emergency measures to be taken when a resident experiences a seizure
- Define the term *chronic brain syndrome*

Key Terminology

- myelin — insulating material that surrounds nerve fibers and is destroyed in multiple sclerosis
- euphoric — experiencing an exaggerated feeling of well-being
- remission — when symptoms decrease or go away completely
- exacerbation — when symptoms return or increase
- quadriplegic — a person with paralysis of all four limbs and the trunk of the body
- paraplegic — a person with paralysis of the lower limbs and lower trunk of the body
- level of injury — the location of a spinal cord injury in relationship to the vertebrae that surround the cord
- proprioception — knowledge of the location of body parts
- flaccid — limp
- hyperactive — overactive
- spasm — a sudden, uncontrolled jerking movement
- atrophy — the wasting away of unused muscles
- credé — applying pressure over the area of the abdomen above the bladder to push the urine out
- hypotension — low blood pressure
- autonomic dysreflexia — a life-threatening emergency that occurs in quadriplegics and results in severe high blood pressure
- cerebral vascular accident (CVA) — a stroke
- thrombosis — the condition of having a blood clot
- embolus — a blood clot that travels from one place in the body to another
- hemiplegia — paralysis of one side of the body
- aphasia — the loss of language
- emotional lability — radical changes in emotion caused by overreaction to a stimulus

- seizure — a sudden attack
- encephalitis — inflammation of the brain
- meningitis — inflammation of the membranes that cover the brain and spinal cord
- grand mal seizure — a type of seizure characterized by loss of consciousness and followed by a convulsion
- convulsion — a sudden, involuntary tightening of the muscles, followed by jerking movements of the arms and legs
- petit mal seizure — a brief seizure with no loss of consciousness that occurs most often in children
- focal or Jacksonian seizures — spasmodic movements of the hands, face, or foot that may spread to other areas of the body
- psychomotor seizure — a temporary impairment of consciousness associated with loss of judgment or abnormal acts
- epilepsy — a condition characterized by seizures with no known cause
- brain syndrome — a number of signs or symptoms that indicate brain disease is present
- orientation — the ability to describe person, place, and time accurately
- reality orientation — a method of reminding residents of reality through a structured class
- validation — a method of acknowledging and accepting the feelings of the disoriented or maloriented resident

Learning Activities

1. Three common symptoms of Parkinson's disease are

   (1) Rigid muscles

   (2) Tremors

   (3) Weakness

2. Nursing care of a resident with Parkinson's disease includes care of the ___Skin___, keeping food ___warm___, taking time to ___listen___, encouraging self-care, walking ___in front___ of the resident who is ambulating, or having the resident push a straight chair or use a pick-up walker.

3. Which age group is most often affected by multiple sclerosis?

   a. Birth to 12 years
   (b) 20 to 40 years
   c. 60 to 80 years
   d. 80 to 100 years

4. In a brief statement, explain why the nature of multiple sclerosis makes adjustment difficult for the victim.

It may come & go for no apparent reason & the pt. cannot not depend upon the fact of a cure.

5. Define the terms *remission* and *exacerbation.*

Remission - symptoms go away

Exacerbation - Symptoms return

6. A Quadriplegic is a person with paralysis of all four extremities and the trunk of the body. A Paraplegic is a person with paralysis of the lower extremities and the lower trunk.

7. Give one effect of spinal cord injury on each of the following systems.

a. The integumentary system – immobility

b. The muscular system - Below level of injury, the Paralyzed muscles will appear thin & lack bulk = wasting away

c. The skeletal system – Weak & porous bones

d. The digestive system – Constipation due to a slower digestive system

e. The urinary system – Kidney & bladder stones

f. The nervous system - Paralysis & loss of sensation

g. The cardiovascular system – low blood pressure, blood clot formation.

h. The respiratory system - risky Pneumonia
shallow breathing, difficulty breathing.

i. The reproductive system - lacking sensation, erection

8. Autonomic dysreflexia is an ___emergency___ situation that threatens the ___life___ of a person with a ___spinal cord___ injury. Stimuli from the skin, the bowel, and the ___bladder___ cause severe ~~dysreflexia~~ high BP. The person develops headache, ___goose pimples___, sweating of the face, and a ___stuffy nose___. The blood pressure ___increases___, and the heart rate ___slows___. One action the nursing assistant can take immediately is to ___elevate___ the head of the bed.

9. Explain the nature of a cerebrovascular accident (CVA), or stroke. Include the following elements:

   a. Factors placing a person at risk for stroke
   b. Definition of stroke
   c. Common symptoms

A stroke is caused by bleeding in the brain or by the existence of a blood clot in a blood vessel of the brain.

High blood pressure is a factor as is arteriosclerosis

frequently the victim is paralyzed on one side of the body.

face - droopy eyelid or inability to close eye.

10. Select a resident who has a diagnosis of stroke, and write a three-page case history. Use blank paper, the chart, the resident, and the family for information. Compare the resident selected to the description in the textbook (pages 284 through 288) and to your answer to question 9.

11. Communication with an aphasic resident can be improved by

(1) Getting their attention.

(2) Talk + work slowly

(3) Use body language | gestures

(4) Writing

12. List three goals of nursing care for a resident with impaired consciousness.

(1) Maintain resident's ability to breathe

(2) Skin care - preventing breakdown

(3) Stimulate the senses

13. Certain conditions can increase the frequency of seizures in a person with epilepsy. List them.

(1) Other illness

(2) lack of physical activity

(3) Fatigue

(4) Constipation

(5) Emotional stress

14. For the following statements about epilepsy, indicate those that are true (*T*) and those that are false (*F*).

__T__ Epilepsy does not affect the intelligence.
__F__ Epilepsy is contagious.
__F__ Epilepsy is painful.
__T__ Epilepsy does not shorten life.
__T__ A person with epilepsy can lead a normal life, including marriage, raising a family, and participating in sports.

15. When a seizure occurs, the major concern is to __protect__ the resident from __injury__. Do not __leave__ the resident. Use the call signal to summon help. Assist the resident to __lie down__ to prevent a fall. Protect the __head__ with a pillow or other soft cushion. Never attempt to __restrain__ the resident from moving. If possible, turn the resident to __one side__ to allow secretions to drain from the mouth and nose. Observe the seizure so you can report the

lengths, the presence of any warning, the part of the body where the seizure began, any incidence of incontinence, and any injury.

16. Define the term *chronic brain syndrome*. Compare it with *acute brain syndrome*. Symptoms are not reversable w/ chronic. Acute - symptoms seem to be tretable & reversable.

Notes

Critical Skill Checklist for Chapter 11, Section 2

◆ Accurately complete the Learning Activities. 11/14 Date 7f Initial

Date of Completion 11-24-00 Instructor Carolyn Moore, RN

SECTION 3 ■ The Resident with Alzheimer's Disease and Dementias of the Alzheimer's Type

Objectives

When you have completed this section, you will be able to

- ◆ Define *Alzheimer's disease*
- ◆ Identify statements about Alzheimer's disease that are true and statements that are false
- ◆ Categorize the symptoms of Alzheimer's disease into the appropriate stages of the disease
- ◆ Identify the three most important considerations when providing care to a resident with Alzheimer's disease
- ◆ List four factors that worsen the behavior in a resident with Alzheimer's disease

Key Terminology

- ◆ Alzheimer's disease — an incurable disease affecting the brain
- ◆ dementia — a condition characterized by the deprivation of reason and by mental deterioration
- ◆ catastrophic reactions — sudden changes from baseline behavior that are socially unacceptable
- ◆ apathy — a lack of feeling or interest in things

Learning Activities

1. What is Alzheimer's disease?

   (a.) An incurable disease affecting the brain

   b. A part of the normal aging process

   c. A reversible condition characterized by loss of memory, loss of orientation, and impaired judgment

   d. A chronic, irreversible condition affecting long-term memory and the ability to learn new skills

2. Indicate which of the following statements about Alzheimer's disease are true (*T*) and which are false (*F*).

   __F__ Alzheimer's is the fourth leading cause of death in the United States in people over 75 years of age.

   __F__ Alzheimer's disease never occurs in anyone under 65 years of age.

   __F__ By the year 2040, one in every three families will be directly touched by this disease.

   __T__ The only accurate way to diagnose Alzheimer's disease is by examining brain tissue after death.

   __F__ Alzheimer's disease affects people in an orderly fashion. They proceed through the first stage, the second stage, and the terminal stage within a three-year period.

3. Next to each symptom of Alzheimer's disease, place a *1* if it occurs in the first stage, a *2* if it occurs in the second stage, and a *3* if it occurs in the terminal stage.

   __2__ May see or hear things that are not there and will be convinced they are real

   __1__ Has poor judgment, makes poor decisions

   __2__ Is unable to remember what he or she was just told to do

   __3__ Loses control of bowel and bladder functions

   __3__ Cannot recognize family or self in a mirror

   __1__ Loses initiative, cannot start anything

   __2__ May become suspicious, irritable, fidgety, silly, or subject to mood swings, especially tears

   __3__ May experience seizures, difficulty swallowing, skin breakdown, or infection

4. The three most important considerations when providing care to a resident with Alzheimer's disease are

(1) They are not deliberately difficult

(2) Trial + error determines what may work w/ Pt.

(3) Remember, it is how the pt. perceives that will trigger behavior

3 C's
1) Caution - Protect.
2) Communication
3) Comfort - Physical, emot. environmental

5. List four factors that worsen the behavior of a resident with Alzheimer's disease.

(1) fatigue

(2) Change of routine or environment

(3) Too much stimulation - (trouble understanding + processing)

(4) Physical pain, Discomfort, + reactions to med.

Notes

Critical Skill Checklist for Chapter 11, Section 3

◆ Accurately complete the Learning Activities. 11/14/00 Date ____ Initial

◆ Do a case study on a resident with Alzheimer's by comparing the resident with the textbook picture of Alzheimer's disease. Attempt to place the resident in the appropriate stage. ____ Date ____ Initial

Date of Completion 11-24-00 Instructor Carolyn Moore, RN

CHAPTER 12

The Respiratory System

SECTION 1 ■ Anatomy and Physiology

Objectives

When you have completed this section, you will be able to

- Define the term *respiration*
- Identify the major function of the lungs
- List three age-related changes that affect the respiratory system

Key Terminology

- respiration — an exchange of gases between an organism and the environment in which it lives. A respiration consists of breathing in and out one time
- alveoli — tiny air sacs in the lungs through which oxygen enters the blood
- metabolism — complex processes of living cells—the work of the cell. Oxygen is used and carbon dioxide is produced
- trachea — the windpipe; the passage through which air moves from the larynx to the bronchi
- bronchi — the two main branches of the trachea
- larynx — the voice box; contains the vocal cords, which make speech possible
- epiglottis — a small piece of cartilage that covers the opening to the trachea
- aspiration — a condition that occurs when small pieces of food, fluid, mucus, or vomitus are taken into the air passages
- diaphragm — a muscular organ that separates the chest and abdominal cavities
- cyanosis — a condition in which the skin, lips, and nail beds become blue-gray or ashen due to lack of oxygen in the circulatory system

Learning Activities

1. What is respiration?
   a. Small amounts of fluid taken into the lungs
   b. Difficulty breathing
   c. A covering over the trachea that prevents aspiration
   d. The process of breathing in and out one time

2. What are the major functions of the lungs?
   (1) Provide H_2O to the cells of the body
   (2) Remove waste products in the form of carbon dioxide.

3. List three age-related changes affecting the respiratory system.
   (1) Respiratory muscles weaken
   (2) Lung tissue becomes less elastic
   (3) Posture - limiting expansion of the chest (stooped)

Notes

Critical Skill Checklist for Chapter 12, Section 1

◆ Accurately complete the Learning Activities.	11/14/00 Date	TJ Initial
◆ Review the anatomical illustration, "The Respiratory System" (Figure 12–1, p. 304 in the text).	Date	Initial

Date of Completion 11-24-00 Instructor Carolyn Moore RN

SECTION 2 ■ The Resident with Respiratory Disease

Objectives

When you have completed this section, you will be able to

- Identify the most important factor contributing to respiratory disease
- Explain why residents confined to bed are at risk for pneumonia
- Describe two nursing measures to prevent pneumonia
- Identify true statements related to providing oxygen therapy

Key Terminology

- pneumonia — an acute inflammation or infection of the lung
- emphysema — a disease in which the bronchioles become plugged with mucus
- asthma — a disease of the bronchi characterized by difficulty breathing, wheezing, and a sense of tightness or constriction in the chest due to muscle spasm
- chronic obstruction pulmonary disease (COPD) — a group of lung diseases, including emphysema, asthma, and chronic bronchitis
- cannula — a plastic tube used to give oxygen to a resident
- humidifier — a container filled with water through which oxygen passes, adding moisture to the air
- postural drainage — draining secretions from the respiratory passages through special positioning
- cilia — small hairlike projections within the respiratory passages
- sputum — a substance collected from the lungs that contains mucus, saliva, and sometimes blood or purulent material
- purulent material — a liquid inflammation product containing cells and other fluid

Learning Activities

1. What is the most important factor contributing to respiratory disease?
   a. Age
   b. Stress
   c. Air pollution
   d. Smoking

2. Residents confined to bed are more likely to develop pneumonia because secretions ___pool___ in the ___lungs___.

3. To prevent pneumonia in the resident confined to bed, the nursing assistant should do which two things?

a. Give oral hygiene

(b.) Reposition frequently

c. Administer oxygen

(d.) Encourage coughing and deep breathing

4. Indicate which of the following statements about oxygen therapy are true (*T*) and which are false (*F*).

T All cells require oxygen.

F The only way to increase the oxygen supply is to breathe deeper.

T A nasal cannula is one way to supply residents with extra oxygen.

T Oxygen should be considered a potential hazard when stored.

F Residents and visitors may smoke when oxygen is in use if they stand three feet away from the oxygen source.

T Some residents may not be able to tolerate too much oxygen.

T The oxygen humidifier should not be allowed to run dry.

T Because oxygen is drying, residents receiving it require additional oral hygiene.

Notes

Critical Skill Checklist for Chapter 12, Section 2

◆ Accurately complete the Learning Activities.

Date 11/14 Initial [initials]

Date of Completion 11-24-00 Instructor Carolyn Moore, RN

CHAPTER 13

The Cardiovascular System

SECTION 1 ■ Anatomy and Physiology

Objectives

When you have completed this section, you will be able to

- ◆ Describe the two basic functions of the cardiovascular system
- ◆ Identify the most important functions of red blood cells and white blood cells
- ◆ Describe the various types of blood vessels
- ◆ Explain why elderly people tire more easily and have less reserve energy than young people
- ◆ Identify the symptoms of three conditions affecting the cardiovascular system

Key Terminology

- ◆ plasma — the fluid portion of the blood
- ◆ platelets — blood cells that are essential to the clotting of blood
- ◆ arteries — blood vessels that carry oxygen-rich blood away from the heart
- ◆ arterioles — tiny arteries that carry blood from the large arteries to the capillaries
- ◆ capillaries — the smallest blood vessels in the circulatory system; they nourish all body cells
- ◆ veins — blood vessels that carry oxygen-poor blood back to the heart, lungs, and kidneys
- ◆ venules — tiny veins that carry blood from the capillaries to the large veins of the body
- ◆ lymph vessels — tiny capillary-like structures that collect lymph from the tissue spaces
- ◆ blood pressure — the measurable force of the blood against the walls of a blood vessel

- ◆ heart — a cone-shaped muscle in the chest that functions as a pump, circulating blood through the blood vessels
- ◆ septum — the tissue that divides that heart into right and left halves
- ◆ right atrium — the chamber on the right side of the heart, which receives oxygen-poor blood from the large veins of the body
- ◆ right ventricle — the chamber on the right side of the heart, which squeezes and pumps blood into the pulmonary artery
- ◆ left atrium — the chamber on the left side of the heart, which receives oxygen-rich blood from the pulmonary veins
- ◆ left ventricle — the chamber on the left side of the heart, which pumps oxygen-rich blood into the aorta
- ◆ pacemaker — the part of the heart that transmits an electrical impulse resulting in the heartbeat
- ◆ electrocardiogram — a device that records the heart's electrical conduction system on a graph for analysis by a physician
- ◆ tricuspid valve — a valve located between the right atrium and the right ventricle
- ◆ pulmonic valve — a valve located between the right ventricle and the pulmonary artery
- ◆ aortic valve — a valve located between the left ventricle and the aorta
- ◆ aorta — the largest artery in the body
- ◆ hypertension — high blood pressure

Learning Activities

1. The two basic functions of the cardiovascular system are to ___Carry___ nutrients and ___H_2O O_2___ to all body ___Cells___ by way of the ___blood vessels___ and to remove ___Waste products___ from the ___Cells___.

2. The most important function of the red blood cells is to carry ___Red blood cells___ from the lungs to the ___Cells___. The most important function of the white blood cells is to fight ___infection___.

3. Match the types of blood vessels in column A with the descriptions in column B.

Column A

b lymph vessels

e arteries

f venules

d capillaries

c veins

a arterioles

Column B

a. very tiny arteries of the body, which carry blood from the larger arteries to the capillaries

b. tiny capillary-like structures that collect lymph

c. blood vessels that carry oxygen-poor blood back to the heart

d. the smallest blood vessels in the circulatory system; they nourish the cells

e. blood vessels that carry oxygen-rich blood away from the heart

f. tiny veins of the body which carry blood from the capillaries to the large veins of the body

4. Explain why elderly people tire more easily and have less reserve energy than young people.

Decreased heart rate, less amount of blood pumped, less cardiac output.

5. Match the conditions in column A with the symptoms in column B.

Column A

b hypertension

c congestive heart failure

a cerebral vascular accident

Column B

a. ruptured blood vessel in the brain

b. high blood pressure

c. fluids backing up into the lungs

Notes

Critical Skill Checklist for Chapter 13, Section 1

	Date	Initial
◆ Accurately complete the Learning Activities.	11/14/00	TJ
◆ Review the anatomical illustration "The Heart and Blood Vessels" (Figures 13–2 and 13–4, pp. 316 and 318 in the text).		

Date of Completion 11-24-00 Instructor Carolyn Moore, RN

SECTION 2 ▪ The Resident with Heart Disease

Objectives

When you have completed this section, you will be able to

- ◆ Identify three types of heart disease and the signs and symptoms associated with each
- ◆ Describe the nursing measures needed when a resident takes nitroglycerine
- ◆ Apply antiembolism stockings
- ◆ Identify three important measures associated with providing care to a resident with an amputation
- ◆ List three guidelines for providing care to a resident with heart disease

Key Terminology

- ◆ cardiovascular insufficiency — a form of heart disease in which there is a decreased blood supply to the major organs of the body
- ◆ arteriosclerosis — the thickening and loss of elasticity in the arteries of the body
- ◆ atherosclerosis — a form of arteriosclerosis in which the arteries become clogged or blocked with various substances
- ◆ plaque — a substance that clogs arteries
- ◆ cardiac bypass surgery — surgery to improve blood circulation throughout the heart muscle and the coronary arteries by replacing the clogged or blocked arteries
- ◆ cardiac angioplasty — a surgical procedure used to open clogged coronary arteries with a special pressurized balloon threaded through the clogged portion of the artery
- ◆ infarct — the death of tissue due to lack of circulation
- ◆ myocardial infarction (MI), heart attack — when part of the heart muscle dies due to inadequate blood supply
- ◆ pacemaker — a mechanical device implanted in the chest wall to substitute for the nonfunctioning or malfunctioning conduction system of the heart
- ◆ angina pectoris — acute chest pain caused by decreased blood supply to the heart
- ◆ congestive heart failure — an abnormal condition characterized by circulatory congestion caused by cardiac disorders
- ◆ peripheral vascular disease — poor circulation, especially in the legs and feet, due to changes in the blood vessels caused by arteriosclerosis
- ◆ stasis ulcers — open wounds or sore on the legs caused by a stoppage of blood flow
- ◆ varicose veins — a type of vascular disease in which the veins are swollen and painful due to loss of elasticity, prolonged standing, and lack of exercise
- ◆ thrombus — a blood clot that frequently obstructs the blood supply
- ◆ embolus — a blood clot that moves within the bloodstream
- ◆ gangrene — a disease that results in the death of tissue due to poor circulation and the presence of certain bacteria
- ◆ amputation — the cutting off of a body part
- ◆ sodium chloride — table salt; usually limited for residents with heart disease

Learning Activities

1. Which type of heart disease is described by each set of signs and symptoms? Write the name of the condition above the list.

   a. Condition: Congestive Heart failure

   - Congestion in the lungs
   - Difficulty breathing
   - Restlessness, anxiety
   - Edema of legs, feet, hands, face
   - Weight gain
   - Weakness, fatigue
   - Dizziness, confusion
   - Chest pain

   b. Condition: Hypertension

   - Faintness or dizziness
   - Headache
   - Difficulty with vision or speech
   - Nosebleed
   - Flushed, red face
   - Sudden changes in behavior, orientation

   c. Condition: Peripheral Vascular disease

   - Edema or swelling of extremities
   - Changes in skin temperature
   - Shiny, dry, flaky skin
   - Pain
   - Absence of pulse in legs and feet

2. Find out which of the residents to whom you are assigned take nitroglycerine. These tiny White Nitroglycerin pills may be kept at bedside, w/pt. They are placed under tongue when the resident experiences Chest pain. It is your responsibility to Observe assist and notify L.N. anytime you see a resident take nitroglycerine.

3. Which of the following nursing measures are associated with providing care to a resident with an amputation?

   a. Encourage maximum independence.
   b. Have a matter-of-fact attitude about the amputation.
   c. Prevent infection.
   d. Protect the stump from injury.
   e. Report any sores, bleeding, or drainage from the wound.

4. List three guidelines for providing care to a resident with heart disease.

(1) Plan & organize care / Balancing activity & rest

(2) Assist pt. w/ following diet ordered by physician.

(3) Be alert of the signs & symptoms of heart disease or change in residents condition.

Notes

Critical Skill Checklist for Chapter 13, Section 2

◆ Accurately complete the Learning Activities. 11/14/00 Date [initial] Initial

◆ Demonstrate applying antiembolism stockings. ______ Date ______ Initial

Date of Completion 11-24-00 Instructor Carolyn Moore, RN

CHAPTER 14

The Endocrine System

SECTION 1 ■ Anatomy and Physiology

Objectives

When you have completed this section, you will be able to

- ◆ Identify the endocrine glands
- ◆ Match the glands with their functions
- ◆ Identify and describe the most common endocrine disease

Key Terminology

- ◆ hormones — fluids secreted by the endocrine glands
- ◆ pituitary gland — the master gland of the body
- ◆ thyroid gland — the largest of the endocrine glands; it produces hormones that regulate growth and the metabolic rate
- ◆ parathyroid glands — a pair of small glands located within the thyroid gland; they produce a hormone that, together with the thyroid, regulates the level of calcium and phosphorous in the body
- ◆ thymus gland — a two lobed, ductless gland that is believed to play a role in the immune system of the body
- ◆ pancreas — a large gland located below and behind the liver and stomach that is both an endocrine and an exocrine gland; the endocrine portion secretes insulin and glucagon, both of which play a role in the level of sugar in the blood
- ◆ adrenal glands — two small, extremely important glands located on the top of each kidney that are involved in the metabolism of proteins, fat, and carbohydrates, influence the levels of sodium and potassium, and are essential to fluid and electrolyte balance; they also produce the hormones that aid the body in reacting to stress

- ovaries — glands in the female that produce ova and at regular intervals produce the hormones estrogen and progesterone, which are essential in the reproductive processes and influence a woman's physical characteristics
- ovulation — the process by which an ovum (egg) is discharged from an ovary at regular intervals
- testes — glands in the male that produce sperm and the hormone testosterone, which is responsible for masculine physical characteristics
- exocrine — producing a secretion that is released externally
- sweat glands — the 2 million small exocrine glands that produce sweat to cool the body and eliminate waste
- salivary glands — exocrine glands in the mouth that secrete saliva, which contains enzymes needed to begin the process of food breakdown
- mammary glands — glandular tissue of the breasts
- bulbo-urethral glands — glands located near the prostrate in males

Learning Activities

1. Identify the following endocrine glands on the diagram of the body in Figure 14-1.

    a. Adrenal
    b. Thymus
    c. Ovaries (in women)
    d. Thyroid
    e. Pituitary
    f. Pancreas
    g. Parathyroid
    h. Testes (in men)

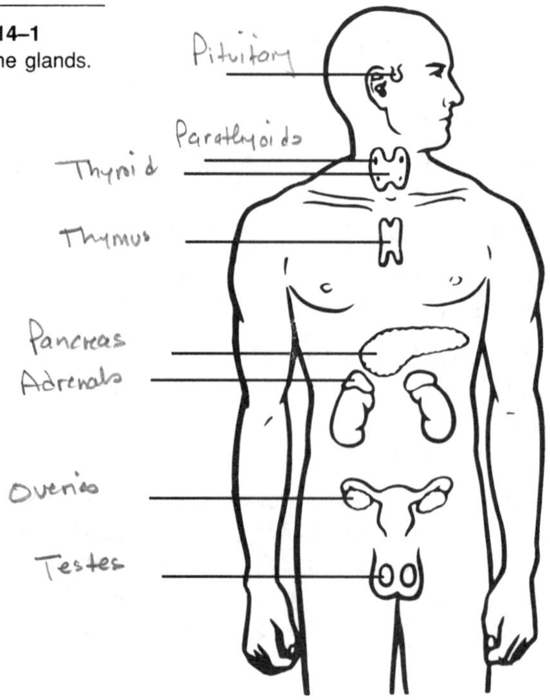

Figure 14–1
Endocrine glands.

2. Match the glands in column A with the functions in column B.

Column A		Column B
e	testes	a. the largest of the endocrine glands; produces hormones that regulate growth and the metabolic rate
f	pancreas	b. is responsible for ovulation and feminine physical characteristics
g	adrenal glands	c. considered the "master" gland; regulates metabolism and stimulates other glands to secrete their hormones
c	pituitary gland	d. secretes substances necessary to begin the process of food breakdown
a	thyroid gland	e. is responsible for producing sperm and masculine physical characteristics
b	ovaries	f. secretes insulin and is both an endocrine and an exocrine gland
d	salivary glands	g. two small glands important in the metabolism of protein, fats, and carbohydrates and in the maintenance of fluid and electrolyte balance
h	sweat glands	h. over two million contained in the skin, the purpose of which is to cool the body and to eliminate waste

3. The most common endocrine disease is diabetes.

Describe this disease in your own words. Include a definition, signs and symptoms, and risk factors of the disease.

is a disorder of carbohydrate metabolism in which the ability to breakdown & use carbohydrates is lost due to disturbances in insulin production

Fatigue
Frequent urination
etc

Notes

Critical Skill Checklist for Chapter 14, Section 1

◆ Accurately complete the Learning Activities.

Date	Initial
11/14/00	[illegible]

Date of Completion 11-24-00 Instructor Carolyn Moore, RN

SECTION 2 ■ Care of the Resident with Diabetes Mellitus

Objectives

When you have completed this section, you will be able to

◆ Describe diabetes mellitus

◆ Define four terms related to diabetes mellitus

◆ List four common complications associated with diabetes mellitus

◆ Describe nursing measures that prevent the complications of diabetes

◆ Explain why the nursing assistant should report what a resident who takes insulin does not eat

Key Terminology

◆ diabetes mellitus — a disorder of carbohydrate metabolism in which the ability to break down and use carbohydrates is lost because of disturbances in insulin production

◆ insulin — a hormone secreted by the pancreas that allows the correct amount of glucose to leave the bloodstream and nourish the cells

◆ glucose — a simple sugar that is an essential nutrient of the cell

- hyperglycemia — having too much glucose in the bloodstream due to too little insulin
- glycosuria — glucose that has "spilled over" to the urine
- acetone — a by-product of the metabolism of fats; a ketone
- ketonuria — the presence of acetone in the urine
- acidosis — a dangerous buildup of ketones in the blood, which may lead to coma and death if untreated
- diabetic coma — a life-threatening condition with elevated blood sugar and acidosis
- diabetic shock or insulin shock — a life-threatening condition in which the blood sugar is too low due to an excess of insulin or an insufficient intake of food
- hypoglycemia — low blood sugar
- aneurysm — a weakened area in a blood vessel that can rupture
- reagent — a substance used in a chemical reaction to determine the presence of another substance
- lancet — a sharp implement used to pierce the skin to obtain a blood sample

Learning Activities

1. What is diabetes mellitus?

   a. A disorder of protein metabolism affecting the structure and composition of the blood vessels

   b. A disease that almost always results in blindness and death

   c. A disorder of carbohydrate metabolism due to disturbances in insulin production, which affects many body systems and has life-threatening complications

   d. A disorder of carbohydrate metabolism in which too much insulin is produced by the pancreas

2. Complete the following statements, which define key terms related to diabetes mellitus.

   a. Hypoglycemia is a condition in which there is __low__ blood sugar.

   b. Hyperglycemia is a condition in which there is __high__ blood sugar.

   c. Diabetic coma results from insufficient __insulin__ or too much __sugar__.

   d. Insulin shock occurs when there is too much __insulin__ or not enough __sugar__.

3. List four common complications associated with diabetes mellitus.

(1) Diabetic shock

(2) Diabetic Coma

(3) hyperglycemia

(4) hypoglycemia

(1) Poor Circulation
(2) Susceptibility to infection
(3) Decreased Ability to heal
(4) Ulceration & gangrene of the Feet

Redness / dryness
Ulceration / sores
Circulation problems
no healing

4. Describe at least one nursing measure designed to prevent each of the four complications listed in the previous question.

(1) Injections

(2) Proper diet

(3) Activity

(4) Testing

check these again

Good Foot Care
Do not trim toenails or cut corns or calluses
Monitor & Report food intake
Report any break in the skin or irritation.

Report skin sores
Promote activity
Report non healing
Good skin care + follow diet plan

5. Explain why the nursing assistant should report what a resident who is receiving insulin does *not* eat.

Because their diet is designed according to their needs. If they do not eat, there is danger due to the lack of sugar, etc that is needed - or the danger of too much sugar

Notes

Critical Skill Checklist for Chapter 14, Section 2

- Accurately complete the Learning Activities.

11/15/00 Date | TJ Initial

Date of Completion 11-24-00 Instructor Carolyn Moore, RN

CHAPTER 15

The Reproductive System and Human Sexuality

SECTION 1 ■ Anatomy and Physiology

Objectives

When you have completed this section, you will be able to

- List the two basic functions of the male and female reproductive systems
- Name the primary sex hormones in the male and female
- List four common symptoms associated with prostatic hypertrophy
- List two age-related changes that may affect the reproductive organs of the elderly female resident
- Give a vaginal douche

Key Terminology

- testes — the primary reproductive organs in the male, located in the scrotum, which produce sperm
- sperm — male reproductive cells, which are released upon ejaculation
- scrotum — a sac, located outside the body and posterior to the penis, that contains the testes
- penis — the primary male sex organ
- testosterone — a male hormone that influences both sexual activity and reproduction
- semen — fluid expelled during the male orgasm, which contains water, nutrients, vitamins, and sperm
- urethra — a tube leading from the bladder to the outside of the body, which in the male, expels both urine and semen

- ◆ benign prostatic hypertrophy — a noncancerous enlargement of the prostate gland
- ◆ prostate gland — a firm, muscular gland that encircles the urethra in the male
- ◆ nocturia — the need to get up at night to urinate
- ◆ transurethral surgery — a procedure used to remove some of the prostate, which is enlarged and squeezing the urethra, causing nocturia, frequency of urination, and painful urination
- ◆ impotence — the loss of sexual function
- ◆ ovaries — the primary reproductive organs of the female, which produce ova, which unite with the sperm of the male to create new life
- ◆ ova (eggs) — the specialized reproductive cells of the female
- ◆ estrogen — the primary sex hormone in the female
- ◆ ovulation — a monthly process that releases an ovum from one ovary into the fallopian tube
- ◆ fallopian tube — a tube through which the ovum passes into the uterus
- ◆ uterus (womb) — the place where the fetus grows during pregnancy
- ◆ fertile — able to become pregnant
- ◆ menstruation — the monthly release of blood and the lining of the uterus that occurs when there is no pregnancy
- ◆ clitoris — the primary female sex organ, capable of enlargement and erection upon stimulation
- ◆ menopause — the ending of menstruation, usually occurring between ages 45 and 55 or when the uterus has been surgically removed
- ◆ vulvitis — inflammation of the vulva or area surrounding the urethral and vaginal openings in the female
- ◆ vaginitis — inflammation of the tissues of the vagina
- ◆ vaginal irrigation or douche — the introduction of a solution into the vaginal canal with an immediate return of the solution by gravity
- ◆ prolapse — when the uterus falls down into the vagina
- ◆ hysterectomy — the surgical removal of the uterus

Learning Activities

1. The two basic functions of the male and female reproductive systems are

   (1) Reproduction

   (2) Pleasure

2. What is the primary sex hormone in the male?

   a. Insulin
   b. Testosterone
   c. Adrenalin
   d. Estrogen

3. What is the primary sex hormone in the female?

   a. Cortisone
   b. Testosterone
   c. Thyroid
   d. Estrogen

4. A male resident with prostatic hypertrophy experiences many symptoms. List four of the symptoms.

   (1) painful urination

   (2) hesitancy

   (3) decreased force of the urinary stream

   (4) frequency of urination

5. Two age-related changes that may affect the reproductive organs of the elderly female resident are

   a. Menopause
   b. Vaginitis
   c. Prostatitis
   d. Prolapse
   e. Hysterectomy

Notes

Critical Skill Checklist for Chapter 15, Section 1

- Accurately complete the Learning Activities. 11/15/00 Date TF Initial
- Review the anatomical illustration, "Reproduction" (Figures 15-1 and 15-2, pp. 339 and 341 in the text). ______ Date ______ Initial
- Demonstrate giving a vaginal douche. ______ Date ______ Initial

Date of Completion 11-24-00 Instructor Carolyn Moore, RN

SECTION 2 ■ Human Sexuality

Objectives

When you have completed this section, you will be able to

- Define the term *sexuality*
- Identify three common myths associated with sex and the elderly
- List three ways the nursing assistant can acknowledge the resident's sexuality while providing care

Key Terminology

- sexuality — the quality of being male or female
- masturbation — sexual self-stimulation

Learning Activities

1. Define the term sexuality in two ways. First, describe what sexuality means to you. Then define it as it was defined in the text.

   The quality of being male or female

   Sexuality could also be the act of affection that is shared between people.

   It can also refer to one's "gender".

2. Indicate which of the following statements about sex and the elderly are fact (*F*) and which are myth (*M*).

F M Old people lose all interest in sex.

T F It takes longer for an older man to achieve an erection.

T F Many older people have no appropriate partner.

F M Older men are not capable of intercourse and cannot father children.

T F Masturbation is a normal means of sexual satisfaction that does not harm the individual.

F M Old people don't care how they look and are not interested in being attractive to the opposite sex.

3. List three ways the nursing assistant can acknowledge residents' sexuality while providing care.

(1) Assist w/ personal hygiene

(2) Consider the residents feelings & need for privacy

(3) Show understanding & acceptance when they show interest & affection for one another

Notes

Critical Skill Checklist for Chapter 15, Section 2

- Accurately complete the Learning Activities.

11/15/00 Date

Initial

Date of Completion 11-24-00 Instructor Carolyn Moore, RN

SECTION 3 ■ Sexually Transmitted Diseases

Objectives

When you have completed this section, you will be able to

- ◆ List six sexually transmitted diseases
- ◆ Describe three measures that help protect against sexually transmitted diseases
- ◆ Match four common diseases with their characteristics

Key Terminology

- ◆ sexually transmitted disease (STD) — a disease passed on through sexual activity
- ◆ genitalia — male or female external reproductive organs
- ◆ congenital — present at birth
- ◆ latent — hidden or undeveloped

Learning Activities

1. List six sexually transmitted diseases.

(1) Vaginitis

(2) Genital Herpes

(3) Chlamydia

(4) Gonorrhea

(5) Syphilis

(6) Hiv

2. Which of the following measures help protect against sexually transmitted diseases?

   a. Knowing the signs and symptoms of STDs
   b. Asking your partner about STDs before engaging in sexual activity
   c. Avoiding multiple sexual partners
   d. Using a condom with spermicide
   e. Showering or bathing after sex

3. Match the diseases in column A with the characteristics in column B.

Column A	Column B
c chlamydia	a. marked by a chancre in the male; may involve a rash, hair loss, or fever
b gonorrhea	b. called *clap* or *drip*; males have painful urination; females may have no symptoms
d herpes genitalis	c. 10 percent of all college students may have it; may cause arthritislike symptoms in males and pelvic inflammatory disease in females
a syphilis	d. no known cure exists; increases the risk of cervical cancer

Notes

Critical Skill Checklist for Chapter 15, Section 3

◆ Accurately complete the Learning Activities.

11/15/00
Date

Initial

Date of Completion 11-24-00 Instructor Carolyn Moore, RN

CHAPTER 16

Developmental Disabilities

SECTION 1 ■ Introduction to Developmental Disabilities

Objectives

When you have completed this section, you will be able to

- Define the term *developmental disability*
- List three causes of developmental disability
- Define the term *mental retardation*
- Describe what is meant by the concept of normalization and give examples of a normalized environment
- Define four terms related to developmental disability

Key Terminology

- developmental disability — a legal term describing a severe, chronic disability
- mental retardation — significantly subaverage general intellectual functioning existing with deficits in adaptive behavior and manifested during the developmental period
- intelligence quotient (IQ) — a score obtained on a standardized test
- prenatal — before birth, either hereditary or occurring during pregnancy
- perinatal — occurring during the birth process
- postnatal — occurring after birth, including illness, accidents, or physical abuse
- cerebral palsy — a developmental disability caused by damage to the brain, resulting in the loss of muscular control of the body
- autism — a developmental disability of unknown cause, resulting in a lack of organization in the functioning of the brain
- epilepsy — a disorder in the electrical functioning of the brain, resulting in various kinds of seizures

- normalization — creating an atmosphere that is as close as possible to that experienced by people who are not mentally retarded
- individual program plan (IPP) — a written plan describing goals, objectives, and action to help each client achieve his or her maximum possible development
- interdisciplinary team (ID team) — a group of skilled professionals that works with the client and family to develop the IPP
- qualified mental retardation professional (QMRP) — the professional who heads the ID team
- functional life skills — the skills that enable an individual to function as independently as possible
- fine motor skills — skills that require the use of the fine muscles, such as those of the hands
- gross motor activities — activities that involve the use of the larger muscles of the body
- sensory-motor activities — activities that involve the use of the senses
- active treatment — a concept requiring an individualized treatment plan that is carried out and reevaluated at least annually

---

Learning Activities

1. Describe in your own words what is meant by the term *developmental disability.*

   It describes a disease of one who has a chronic disability.
   It could mean physical or mental or both.
   Mostly it is evidenced before the age of 22 & it cause physical limitations.

   Compare your definition with the definition on page 349 of the text. If necessary, rewrite your definition in accordance with the text.

2. List the three categories used to describe the causes of developmental disabilities, and give one example of each.

(1) Prenatal - hereditary or during pregnancy
Down Syndrome

(2) Perinatal - during birth process.
oxygen supply is cut off.

(3) Postnatal - after birth -
abuse, accident etc

3. What is mental retardation?

a. A severe chronic disability manifested before the person attains twenty-two years

b. A disability that results from a lack of organization in the functioning of the brain

c. Significantly sub-average general intellectual functioning existing with deficits in adaptive behavior and manifested before the person attains twenty-two years

d. A disorder in the electrical functioning of the brain, resulting in various kinds of seizures

4. Describe the concept of normalization.

Creating an atmosphere that is as close as possible to the atmosphere provided for those who are not mentally retarded.

Give an example of a normalized environment.

Clothing and grooming.

pg. 352

a work (job) environment to exercise skills.

Treat with Dignity & Respect
Do not exert undue power over Residents
Staff play role of assistant, not parent
Residents encouraged to do all they can for themselves.

5. Match the terms in column A with the definitions in column B.

Column A	Column B
b developmental model	a. based on chronological age, not developmental or mental age
c active treatment	b. based on the belief that all human beings have potential
a age-appropriate	c. requires an individualized plan that is carried out as written and reevaluated annually
d least restrictive alternative	d. an environment that allows the maximum use of skills and the most personal freedom

Notes

Critical Skill Checklist for Chapter 16, Section 1

◆ Accurately complete the Learning Activities. 11/15/00 Date ___ Initial

Date of Completion 11-24-00 Instructor Carolyn Moore, RN

SECTION 2 ■ Behavior Management Principles and Techniques

Objectives

When you have completed this section, you will be able to

◆ Describe the ABCs of behavior modification

◆ Define the terms *fading*, *prompting*, and *shading*

◆ List the three components of graduated guidance

◆ Give examples of verbal, gestural, and physical prompts

◆ Identify types of reinforcers that are appropriate for the nursing assistant to use

Key Terminology

- ◆ behavior — a manner of acting
- ◆ behavior modification — the process of changing behavior patterns by eliminating ineffective behaviors and teaching effective behaviors
- ◆ reinforcer — anything that causes behavior to be repeated and strengthened
- ◆ behavior shaping — the process of creating a new set of behaviors
- ◆ modeling — demonstrating or showing how to behave or how to perform a skill
- ◆ graduated guidance — providing the least amount of assistance or prompting necessary
- ◆ shadowing — a method of giving guidance by keeping the staff member's hands within one inch of the client's hands while following the performance of the skill
- ◆ fading — the process of gradually decreasing the amount of guidance given
- ◆ forward chaining — breaking down a complex skill into specific steps and teaching each step in the order in which it would normally be completed
- ◆ backward chaining — teaching the last step in a complex skill first, then the next to last, and so on
- ◆ aversive — unpleasant or painful
- ◆ advocate — a person who acts to protect the interests of others

Learning Activities

1. List the ABC's of behavior modification, and give an example of each.

   (A) Antecedent - the event occurring before the target behavior.

   (B) behavior -

   (C) Consequent - Result of the behavior.

2. Match the terms in column A with the definitions in column B.

Column A	Column B
b fading	a. the process of creating a new set of behaviors
c prompting	b. the gradual decrease in the amount of guidance
a shaping	c. may be verbal, gestural, or physical

3. List the three components of graduated guidance.

(1) full graduate guidance.

(2) ~~Shadowing~~ Verbal prompting

(3) ~~fading~~ partial graduate guidance (shadowing)

4. For each of the following types of prompts, give one example.

a. Verbal – Praise

b. Gestural - smiles, hands down,

c. Physical - touch, hugs, pats

5. Give examples of reinforcers that a nursing assistant can use to reinforce desirable behavior.

Rewards → Primary - food, drinks
Social = Praise
Physical - Hugs

Notes

Critical Skill Checklist for Chapter 16, Section 2

◆ Accurately complete the Learning Activities.

11/15/00
Date

Y
Initial

Date of Completion 11-24-00 Instructor Carolyn Moore, RN

CHAPTER 17

The Restorative Nursing Assistant

SECTION 1 ■ Roles and Responsibilities of a Restorative Nursing Assistant

Objectives

When you have completed this section, you will be able to

- ◆ Explain why health promotion and prevention of disease are essential to an LTC facility's restorative program
- ◆ Describe the overall philosophy of a restorative nursing program
- ◆ Identify tasks that would be performed by a restorative nursing assistant
- ◆ Write a restorative weekly summary, using measurable, behavioral terms, from information provided

Key Terminology

- ◆ rehabilitation — the restoration of an individual to the fullest physical, mental, social, vocational, and economic capacity of which he or she is capable

Learning Activities

1. Explain why health promotion and prevention of disease are essential to an LTC facility's restorative program.

of the long term nature of care & the prevention of disease.

2. Describe the overall philosophy of a restorative nursing program.

Return the resident to the fullest level of existence
Physical
mental
Social etc

3. On the following list, mark an X by the tasks generally performed by the restorative nursing assistant.

- __X__ Teaching residents transfer techniques
- _____ Passing fresh ice water daily
- _____ Performing daily personal hygiene tasks
- __X__ Charting weekly the residents' response or lack of response to established goals
- __X__ Working closely with the physical therapist
- _____ Feeding residents
- __X__ Providing assistance/training in activities of daily living
- __X__ Working with other nursing personnel to ensure that residents are properly positioned

4. From the following information, write a weekly summary using measurable, behavioral terms.

Restorative order: Walk resident daily with RNA to improve strength and balance.

Problem: Res. weak following bed rest for pneumonia. Unsteady on feet, balance poor.

Approach: RNA to amb. daily. Increase distance. NA to stand res. at bedside q shift and walk with res. to bathroom as needed.

Goal: Improved balance and increased strength through daily ambulation with RNA. Amb. with minimal assistance of one by ____________________ (date).

Daily Notes

Monday notes: Resident was unsteady and required assistance of two nursing assistants to stand; walked only distance from bed to door of room with two nursing assistants.

Tuesday notes: Resident refused to walk today; stated, "I feel light-headed today. I'll feel better tomorrow." Reported refusal to charge nurse.

Wednesday notes: Resident more steady, able to stand at bedside with minimal assistance of one nursing assistant. Ambulated to door and into hallway and back to bed, about 40 feet; balance improving. Had to remind her frequently to look forward instead of down.

Thursday notes: Standing at bedside with only standby assistance. Walked with safety belt to nursing station and back—approximately 60 feet. Balance continues to improve, and gait was more even.

Friday notes: Seems a little tired today—balance good, but endurance reduced; only able to ambulate about halfway to nursing station. Stated, "I didn't sleep very well last night."

Saturday notes: Standing at bedside independently, ambulating with steady gait to nursing station, into dayroom, and back to room, with standby assistance only.

Weekly Summary

Over the past, has progressed From assistance of Two To ambulating with steady gait To the Nursing Station and back To Room with Standby assistant only. Balance has improved, but Residents demonstrates poor endurance when She indicates She hasn't Slept well.

Notes

Critical Skill Checklist for Chapter 17, Section 1

- Accurately complete the Learning Activities. 11/15/00 Date — TY Initial
- Review the job description for an RNA in your facility. ______ Date — ______ Initial

Date of Completion 11-24-00 Instructor Carolyn Moore RN

Section 2 ■ Restorative Nursing Procedures

Objectives

When you have completed this section, you will be able to

- Demonstrate teaching a resident to perform range-of-motion exercises independently
- Demonstrate teaching a resident to transfer independently
- Identify true statements regarding achieving balance and increasing strength for ambulation
- Demonstrate special positioning techniques to prevent pressure, contractures, and foot drop
- Demonstrate the correct procedure for giving a whirlpool bath
- Explain why performing activities of daily living (ADLs) independently is an important goal for most residents whose functional abilities have been lost or are impaired

Key Terminology

- supervision — the presence of a staff member to provide encouragement and verbal guidance
- standby assistance — the presence of a staff member to observe and be readily available if help is needed.
- minimum assistance — when the resident performs about 75 percent of the tasks and the nursing assistant performs the remaining 25 percent
- moderate assistance — when the resident performs about 50 percent of the tasks and the nursing assistant performs the other 50 percent
- maximum assistance — when the resident performs about 25 percent of the tasks and the nursing assistant performs 75 percent

Learning Activities

1. Place an *X* in the space next to each true statement regarding achieving balance and increasing strength for ambulation.

   __X__ Ambulation has positive effects on body systems.

   __X__ To be ready to ambulate, the resident needs both strength and balance.

   ______ Ambulation decreases muscle strength.

   ______ The nursing assistant will be able to determine when a resident is ready for ambulation.

   __X__ To protect yourself and the resident from injury, you will need to practice good body mechanics.

   __X__ The first time a resident ambulates after a period of illness is very important in building confidence and increasing motivation.

2. Performing ADLs independently is an important goal for most residents whose functional abilities have been lost or are impaired. Explain why.

   So they will not feel humiliated/dependent

Notes

Critical Skill Checklist for Chapter 17, Section 2

◆ Accurately complete the Learning Activities.	11/15/00 Date	JJ Initial
◆ Demonstrate teaching a resident to perform range-of-motion exercises independently.	✓ Date	Initial
◆ Demonstrate teaching a resident to transfer independently.	✓ Date	Initial
◆ Demonstrate special positioning techniques to prevent pressure, contractures, and foot drop.	✓ Date	Initial
◆ Demonstrate giving a whirlpool bath.	✓ Date	Initial

Date of Completion 11-24-00 Instructor Carolyn Moore, RN

CHAPTER 18

Subacute and Emergency Care in the Long-Term Care Facility

SECTION 1 ■ Subacute Services

Objectives

When you have completed this section, you will be able to

- ◆ Identify the types of services provided in a subacute unit
- ◆ Explain why the nursing assistant in a subacute unit must be very well trained

Key Terminology

- ◆ subacute services — the advanced medical services provided in a designated part of a long-term care facility
- ◆ medical subacute — treatments and services for patients with complex medical needs
- ◆ intensive rehabilitation programs — physical, occupational, and speech therapies provided at the maximum pace tolerated by the patient

Learning Activities

1. Identify the types of services provided in a subacute unit.

IV's
Post operative Care (fractures etc)
Complex wound Care
Tracheotomy

Head injuries
Ventelator
Respitory
Spec. Oncology Care

2. Why must the nursing assistant in a subacute unit be very well trained?

There are specialized care patients. Medical needs are complex aggressive needs

Notes

Critical Skill Checklist for Chapter 18, Section 1

- Accurately complete the Learning Activities. 11/15/00 Date TJ Initial

Date of Completion 11-24-00 Instructor Carolyn Moore, RN

SECTION 2 ■ Care of the Subacute Patient

Objectives

When you have completed this section, you will be able to

- Identify true statments related to infusion therapy
- List four important observations that should be reported to the charge nurse immediately when providing care to a patient with an intravenous line
- Describe the primary role of the nursing assistant in providing care to a patient with an intravenous line or a port-a-cath
- Explain why the nursing assistant must report any changes of condition to the charge nurse immediately when caring for a resident with a head or brain injury

- Identify five specific nursing actions that promote wound healing
- List the signs of respiratory distress that should be reported immediately to the licensed nurse when caring for a patient with a tracheostomy

---

Key Terminology

- peripherally inserted catheter (PICC line or port-a-cath) — a surgically implanted catheter that allows for repeated use of an injection site
- patient-controlled analgesic pump (PCA) — a mechanical device that controls the amount of medication so that a continuous dosage can be received; it allows the patient to self-administer additional intermittent dosages as prescribed by the physician
- wound — a disruption in the continuity and regulatory process of tissue cells
- first intention healing — when wounds are surgically closed and dressed to promote healing
- second intention healing — when wounds are left open due to infection and are allowed to drain to promote healing
- tracheostomy — a surgical opening made into the trachea to provide the patient with an artificial airway

---

Learning Activities

1. Place an *X* in the space next to each true statement related to infusion therapy.

   _____ Intravenous infusions are used only to deliver certain medications.

   __X__ Intravenous infusions are usually delivered through a pump or a rate-controlled device.

   _____ The patient with an intravenous infusion must be confined to bed.

   _____ The nursing assistant should reconnect as quickly as possible any IV tubing that is disconnected.

   __X__ The type, amount, and rate of infusion is ordered by the physician.

2. List four important observations that should be reported immediately to the charge nurse when providing care to a patient with an intravenous line.

   (1) alarms on pump

   (2) Changes in flow or empty bag/bottle

   (3) Fever

   (4) Fluid or blood on floor/bed

3. What is the primary role of the nursing assistant in providing care to a patient with an intravenous line or a port-a-cath?

To be sure it is not being pulled

4. When caring for a resident with a head or brain injury, the nursing assistant must report any change in condition to the charge nurse immediately. Explain why.

Due to Rapid change + it is/could be an emergency + life threatening – Vitals must be taken

5. List five specific nursing actions that promote wound healing.

(1) adequate nutrition + hydration

(2) Abscence of Pressure to enhance circulation

(3) Good skin hygene

(4) Good Physciological health

(5) " Psychological "

6. List the signs of respiratory distress that should be reported immediately to the licensed nurse when caring for a patient with a tracheostomy.

(1) Difficulty in breathing
(2) Rattling sounds
(3) Bubbling secretions or blood from trache site
(4) Cyanosis
(5) Breathing increase / decrease

Notes

Critical Skill Checklist for Chapter 18, Section 2

- ◆ Accurately complete the Learning Activities.

  ____________ Date ____________ Initial

- ◆ Demonstrate changing the gown of a patient with an IV.

  ____________ Date ____________ Initial

Date of Completion 11-24-00 Instructor Carolyn Moore, RN

SECTION 3 ▪ Basic Emergency Care

Objectives

When you have completed this section, you will be able to

- ◆ Describe the goal of providing first aid
- ◆ Describe a precaution to take when checking for life-threatening injuries
- ◆ Identify six major changes in respiratory function that signal that a respiratory emergency exists
- ◆ Identify true statements related to complete airway obstruction and the Heimlich maneuver
- ◆ List three signs of cardiac arrest

Key Terminology

- ◆ apnea — the temporary cessation of breathing
- ◆ ambu bag — a ventilating device
- ◆ stridor — a high-pitched sound caused by spasm of the larynx
- ◆ artifical ventilation — rescue breathing
- ◆ Heimlich maneuver — abdominal thrusts delivered in rapid succession to dislodge a foreign object in the airway
- ◆ sternum — the breastbone
- ◆ Tongue-jaw lift — holding the lower jaw and tongue so the mouth cannot close during finger sweeps to remove foreign objects from the mouth
- ◆ cardiopulmonary resuscitation (CPR) — an emergency procedure used to restore circulation and oxygenation when heart, lung, and certain brain functions have stopped
- ◆ clinical death — when breathing has stopped and the heart has ceased beating
- ◆ biological death — when body cells die as a result of the lack of circulation

Learning Activities

1. What is the goal of providing first aid?

   To prevent death
   further injury

2. When checking for life-threatening injuries, do so without Moving the victim because a Spinal injury may be made worse during emergency treatment.

3. List six major changes in respiratory function that signal that a respiratory emergency exists.

   (1) no chest movements or uneven
   (2) no air exchange can be heard or felt
   (3) Breathing is difficult
   (4) Blue/grey color or ashen
   (5) Breathing too fast/slow
   (6) Respirations very shallow or noisy

4. Place an *X* in the space next to each true statement related to complete airway obstruction and the Heimlich maneuver.

   X It is important to determine whether complete or partial airway obstruction is present.
   X Continue efforts until an obstruction is cleared and the resident's airway is open.
   X Position your fist below the rib cage.
   X Give six to ten abdominal thrusts in rapid succession.

5. What are the three signs of cardiac arrest?

   (1) unresponsive
   (2) lack of breathing
   (3) lack of pulse

Notes

Critical Skill Checklist for Chapter 18, Section 3

◆ Accurately complete the Learning Activities.

11/15/00 Date

[illegible] Initial

Date of Completion 11-24-00 Instructor Carolyn Moore, RN

Student Name ______________________________

Date of Enrollment ____________

Critical Skill Checklist

Chapter/Section	Critical Skill	Date	Instructor's Signature
2-1	Demonstrate applying a soft protective device.		
2-1	Demonstrate lifting an object using proper body mechanics.		
2-3	Demonstrate hand-washing procedures.		
2-3	Demonstrate linen-handling procedures.		
2-4	Demonstrate applying a mask and gown.		
2-5	Demonstrate operating a bed and using side rails.		
2-5	Demonstrate making an occupied bed.		
4-4	Demonstrate weighing a resident using a standing scale.		
4-4	Demonstrate weighing a resident using a mechanical scale.		

Chapter/Section	Critical Skill	Date	Instructor's Signature
4-4	Demonstrate weighing a resident using a bed scale.		
4-4	Demonstrate measuring a resident's height using a measuring tape.		
4-4	Demonstrate measuring oral, rectal, and axillary temperatures using a glass thermometer.		
4-4	Demonstrate measuring oral, rectal, and axillary temperatures using a battery-operated electronic thermometer.		
4-4	Demonstrate measuring temperature using an ear-probe thermometer.		
4-4	Demonstrate measuring a resident's pulse.		
4-4	Demonstrate measuring a resident's respirations.		
4-4	Demonstrate measuring a resident's blood pressure.		
6-3	Demonstrate giving a complete bed bath.		
6-3	Demonstrate giving a back rub.		
6-3	Demonstrate giving perineal care.		
6-3	Demonstrate giving a tub bath.		
6-3	Demonstrate giving a shower.		
6-4	Demonstrate brushing the teeth of a dependent resident.		

Chapter/Section	Critical Skill	Date	Instructor's Signature
6-4	Demonstrate caring for dentures.		
6-4	Demonstrate trimming fingernails or toenails.		
6-4	Demonstrate caring for a resident's hair.		
6-4	Demonstrate shaving a resident's beard.		
6-4	Demonstrate dressing a resident who is in bed.		
6-4	Demonstrate dressing a resident who is paralyzed on one side.		
7-3	Demonstrate moving a resident using a lift sheet.		
7-3	Demonstrate moving a resident up in bed with his or her help.		
7-3	Demonstrate turning a resident away from and toward you.		
7-3	Demonstrate turning a resident using the log-rolling technique.		
7-4	Demonstrate transferring a resident using the pivot technique.		
7-4	Demonstrate transferring a dependent resident.		
8-2	Demonstrate performing range-of-motion exercises for a dependent resident.		
8-2	Demonstrate ambulating a resident using the step-by-step procedure.		

Chapter/Section	Critical Skill	Date	Instructor's Signature
8-2	Demonstrate positioning a dependent resident in a wheelchair.		
8-2	Demonstrate positioning a dependent resident in the supine and a semisupine positions.		
8-2	Demonstrate positioning a dependent resident in the prone and semiprone positions.		
9-2	Demonstrate calculating the percentage of food eaten on ten different trays.		
9-3	Demonstrate fastening an internal feeding tube to a resident's clothing.		
9-4	Demonstrate feeding a dependent resident.		
9-5	Demonstrate inserting a rectal suppository.		
9-5	Demonstrate administering a cleansing enema.		
9-5	Demonstrate changing a colostomy bag.		
9-5	Demonstrate collecting a stool specimen.		
10-3	Demonstrate placing a resident on a bedpan.		
10-3	Demonstrate offering a urinal to a male resident.		
10-3	Demonstrate giving perineal care to a resident with a catheter.		

Chapter/Section	Critical Skill	Date	Instructor's Signature
13-2	Demonstrate applying antiembolism stockings.		
15-1	Demonstrate giving a vaginal douche.		
17-3	Demonstrate teaching a resident to perform range-of-motion exercises independently.		
17-3	Demonstrate teaching a resident to transfer independently.		
17-3	Demonstrate special positioning techniques to prevent pressure, contractures, and foot drop.		
17-3	Demonstrate giving a whirlpool bath.		

Preparing for the Competency Evaluation

■ The Competency Evaluation

Under the regulations developed to implement the Omnibus Budget Reconciliation Act (OBRA) of 1987, nursing assistants working in long-term care must be evaluated for competency. This evaluation includes both a written examination and a skill demonstration.

The written evaluation is made up of about seventy-five multiple-choice questions. Each question is followed by four possible answers. Only one is the correct answer.

Although you are preparing for both examinations throughout your training program, there are ways you can improve your test scores and ensure that you will pass.

Attitude

The most important aspect of preparing for the test is your attitude. You must believe in yourself and what you have learned. An "I Can" attitude is key to your success.

Preparation

You have been studying throughout your course, so all you should need now is a review. Use the objectives at the beginning of each lesson in the textbook to review. You will find sample test questions later in this section so you can test yourself. Next to a positive attitude, preparation is the best guarantee of passing the examination.

To increase your score on the written examination, be sure you read each question thoroughly and follow the instructions. Look for qualifying words like *not*, *except*, *rarely*, or *seldom*. Two of the four possible answers can usually be eliminated immediately. That leaves two from which to choose. When selecting your answer, it is usually wise to remember what you were taught, not necessarily what you see being done on a daily basis. In other words, most tests are written to portray the ideal situation. This is the time your experience may get in the way of identifying the right answer. For example, consider this question: "Restraints must be released at least once every __________." The choices may be "a. hour, b. two hours, c. half hour, or d. four hours." Remember that your textbook says every two hours, even though you might think that every hour sounds better. If you are struggling with a particular question, skip it and return later. If you spend too much time on one question, you may never get to several others. Take the time to work through some of the sample questions and the exercise in following instructions that you will find on the following pages.

Physical Preparation

Be sure to get a good night's sleep before your examination. Plan to take the night off from studying. If you try to study up to the last minute, you will feel more pressure, and you will probably be confused. Use the night before to relax and do something that distracts you from the test. You might want to go out with friends or take in a movie. However, do not stay out late or overindulge in alcohol.

On the morning of the test, get up a little early so you are not rushed. Be sure to eat breakfast. If you do not know exactly where you are going to take the test, check it out in advance and plan ahead. People who are late are not admitted into the examination.

Wear comfortable clothing. Bring a sweater or jacket in case the testing room is cold.

■ Are You Paying Attention?

Using the area below, follow these instructions.

1. Read all instructions carefully before beginning.

2. Write your name in the upper right-hand corner.

3. Draw a large circle in the center of the page.

4. Place a smaller circle inside the large circle.

5. To the right of the large circle, draw a triangle.

6. Draw a star to the left of the large circle.

7. Above the large circle, place a large triangle.

8. To the left of the large circle, draw a triangle just like the one in number 5.

9. Draw a bow under the large circle.

10. Follow the instructions for numbers 1 and 2 only. Do not do the others.

■ Sample Questions

Circle the letter preceding the correct answer to each of the following sample questions. Remember to use the process of elimination to help you select the correct response.

1. As death approaches, the last sense to be lost is

   a. taste
   b. hearing
   c. touch
   d. sight

2. Which of the following is not a sign of approaching death?

   a. increased pulse and fever
   b. increased pain and blood pressure
   c. loss of consciousness
   d. slowed and intermittent respirations

3. Mrs. Stubborn does not want to attend bingo this afternoon. This is her right to

   a. privacy
   b. freedom from abuse and neglect
   c. personal choice
   d. none of the above

4. As you are preparing to give Mr. Clean a tub bath, you measure the temperature of the water. It is 114 degrees F. You should

   a. turn on the hot water to increase the temperature to 115 degrees
   b. assist Mr. Clean into the tub
   c. add cold water to decrease the temperature to 105 degrees
   d. have Mr. Clean check the temperature with his hand; if he says it is OK, assist him into the tub

5. When you perform range-of-motion exercises, you should do all of the following except

   a. support the limb being exercised
   b. move the joint slowly and gently through the normal range of motion
   c. exercise past the point of pain
   d. report any reddened or swollen joints to the nurse

As you answered these questions, did you notice in question 2 the word *not*? This is an example of a qualifying word that you will need to watch for when you take the written examination. Another example is in question 5, where the qualifying word is *except*. This one word changes the entire meaning of the question and, of course, the correct answer.

Answers

1. b.
2. b.
3. c.
4. c.
5. c.